THE WRINKLE-FREE ZONE

Your Guide to Perfect Skin in 30 Days

JAMES P. MESCHINO, D.C., M.S.

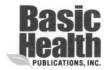

Basic Health
PUBLICATIONS, INC.

The information contained in this book is based upon the research and personal and professional experiences of the author. It is not intended as a substitute for consulting with your physician or other healthcare provider. Any attempt to diagnose and treat an illness should be done under the direction of a healthcare professional.

The publisher does not advocate the use of any particular healthcare protocol but believes the information in this book should be available to the public. The publisher and author are not responsible for any adverse effects or consequences resulting from the use of the suggestions, preparations, or procedures discussed in this book. Should the reader have any questions concerning the appropriateness of any procedures or preparation mentioned, the author and the publisher strongly suggest consulting a professional healthcare advisor.

The author of this book has a financial interest in some of the brand-name products mentioned herein. This does not constitute an endorsement by Basic Health Publications, Inc.

Basic Health Publications, Inc.
8200 Boulevard East
North Bergen, NJ 07047
1-201-868-8336

Library of Congress Cataloging-in-Publication Data
Meschino, James P., 1954–
    The wrinkle-free zone : your guide to perfect skin in 30 days /
James P. Meschino.
        p. cm.
    Includes bibliographical references and index.
    ISBN 1-59120-124-1
    1. Skin—Care and hygiene. 2. Dietary supplements.
3. Skin—Diseases—Alternative treatment. I. Title.

    RL87.M57 2004
    646.7'26—dc22
                                        2004000720

Editor: Susan Davis
Typesetter/Book design: Gary A. Rosenberg
Cover design: Mike Stromberg

Printed in the United States of America

10   9   8   7   6   5   4   3   2   1

Contents

To my family, for their love and support.

My mother, Lena, impressed upon me the virtues of patience, kindness, and compassion for others. She always encouraged me to follow my own path.

My father, Armand, by his own example, taught me the importance of self-discipline, perseverance, and generosity toward others.

My sister, Arlene, has been my guiding light since childhood. She was the first to teach me to believe in myself.

And my brother, Paul, has served, through his seminars and daily life, as a constant reminder of the importance and power of extending unconditional love to others.

Acknowledgments

I would like to thank the many individuals who have assisted me in researching this important subject and aided in the creation and editing of this book, including:

Bruce Cole and his staff—Delia Carnide and Candace and Donna Lundrigan—who helped prepare the original manuscript.

My editor, Susan E. Davis, for her wonderful ability to translate much of my scientific garble into interesting, understandable, entertaining, and usable information.

Bruno Suppa, for his many years of committed effort to the work we have done to help others benefit from evidence-based natural therapies. His own life has served as a testimonial and inspiration to so many people who have been touched by his story and courage.

Carol and Henry Kriegel, who recommended my work to Basic Health Publications.

Arlene Walker and Deborah Worobec, who helped with the design and follow-up of case studies presented in this book, as well as other research activities.

Sharon Kerr and Karen Green, who were the first skin-care professionals to acknowledge my work in nutrition and skin-care management, and who have helped alert hundreds of their colleagues to the importance of these interventions. These two women are also credited with introducing me to the research on the anti-aging and therapeutic effects of encapsulated hyaluronic acid (HA) on the skin, as well as the application of oil of oregano in the management of certain skin conditions.

Pat Lam, who was instrumental in making me a sought-after speaker at skin-care conferences throughout the United States and Canada.

The rest of our office staff—Lisa Anderson, Dina Colangleo, and Kathryn Thomas—who help with all the daily tasks that enable me to get on with my work as a writer, educator, and researcher.

Welcome to the Wrinkle-Free Zone

I t is with great pleasure and anticipation that I introduce you to *The Wrinkle-Free Zone,* a resource that will do much more than help you to prevent or reduce wrinkles. I designed the skin-care program detailed in this book to help you make your skin smooth, soft, supple, and healthy—and not just on your face, hands, and arms, but all over your body.

By following the Wrinkle-Free Zone Program, you will achieve a definite improvement in your skin's texture and appearance. Your skin will also function better and work in greater harmony with your entire body, even helping you to avoid and resist disease. And although you will not be able to see what is happening within the deeper layers of your skin, those cells will be operating at optimal efficiency to provide your skin's surface with the important nutrients it needs to function at its best.

NUTRIENTS ARE NEEDED FOR GOOD SKIN

This book is based on recent scientific discoveries that highlight an extremely important fact about skin care: a radiant, clear, beautiful complexion depends greatly upon the delivery of vital nutrients through the bloodstream to developing cells that lie deep within the skin.

Although we'll delve later into more detail about the importance of proper nutrition to healthy skin, let's begin by noting that growing skin cells extract from the bloodstream specific vitamins, minerals, and other vital nutritional elements. The cells need these nutrients so they can develop and mature into strong, perfectly formed skin cells that will eventually work their way up to the front lines on the skin's surface. There, these emerging cells will be battle-tested by outside forces like wind, chemicals, rain, and sunlight, and through it all they must remain prepared to withstand attacks that could cause disease. Besides helping skin cells resist the elements, ample nutrients are also crucial in giving the skin the structural strength to prevent the wrinkles and age spots that contribute to premature aging.

Deficiencies Hurt the Skin

If your skin is not getting the nutrition it needs, problems result. Medical literature has documented that deficiencies of various vitamins and minerals lead to a variety of skin lesions and disorders. The same literature also confirms that supplementing your diet with the missing nutrients will correct these conditions, usually within a relatively short period of time. The discovery of diseases directly related to vitamin deficiencies, including beriberi, pellagra, scurvy, and others—all with their own characteristic skin lesions—has long provided definitive proof that optimal quantities of vitamins and other nutrients are essential to the skin's health and appearance. Anything less can prevent the skin from attaining its full potential for softness, smoothness, moisture, elasticity, and hydration, and impair its ability to resist the formation of wrinkles, age-related degeneration, and atrophy.

Optimizing the Supply of Nutrients to Skin Cells

Many people believe that the true secret to a beautiful complexion lies in the bottles and jars lining cosmetic and beauty department shelves in stores across the country. Sadly, these individuals are mistaken. Even with topical lotions and anti-aging skin creams and treatments—many of which provide some beneficial effects—the texture and appearance of the skin can never reach its ultimate potential for beauty and anti-aging defense without the optimal supply of healthful nutrients to skin cells from the inside-out. This fact has been the missing link in skin-care management through the years, and it is only now beginning to be appreciated by skin-care professionals and by the public at large.

In general, dermatologists, plastic surgeons, and estheticians have not received extensive formal education or training in nutritional biochemistry and nutritional pharmacology (the use of nutritional supplements at levels exceeding those that food alone can normally provide) as related to skin cell development and maturation, as well as nutritional management of skin conditions. As a result, they often fail to include proper nutrition and supplementation as part of their treatment programs, which is most unfortunate for their patients and clients. However, times are changing.

As a speaker at many international conferences and national workshops attended by skin-care professionals, I am continually amazed by the number of practitioners to whom I have first introduced the role of essential oils, vitamins, and minerals in skin-care management. For the most part, these estheticians and doctors are extremely grateful for this information, and for the scientific references that allow them to further their own investigations into using nutrition and supplementation effectively in the treatment of their clients and patients. Consequently, they are beginning to include these strategies in their skin-care management and anti-aging programs. Nevertheless, old habits generally die hard, and people are not always keen on making changes, so it may take some time before every skin-care professional is armed with the appropriate scientific training to incorporate these proven nutritional methods into practice with every patient.

As a result of these education programs, skin-care professionals are learning that the right combination and dosage of specific vitamins, minerals, and essential oils has been the missing link in building and maintaining healthy skin. It's been one of the best-kept secrets in the health and beauty world for many years. This is not news, however, to those of us involved in the science of nutritional biochemistry, nutritional pharmacology, and natural medicine. The knowledge and application of supplementation with fats, vitamins, and minerals to favorably affect skin texture and skin conditions dates back to the early 1980s, when studies about essential fats and prostaglandin hormones started appearing in clinical and experimental research journals. Many of us have been using these nutritional interventions with our patients for more than twenty years with great success.

Perfect Skin from the Inside-out

Optimal levels of specific nutrients must be available in the bloodstream to properly nourish and support developing skin cells to maturity. Likewise, the successful management of most skin conditions requires, at the very least, complementary dietary and nutritional supplementation in addition to conventional topical treatments. And in order to achieve smoother, softer, moister, and more radiant skin, it's absolutely mandatory for you to take optimal dosages of those nutrients that are known to promote healthy skin.

The Wrinkle-Free Zone offers you a proven system that will enable you to feed your skin the nutrients it needs to improve its texture and appearance, slow its aging, and help prevent and reverse wrinkle formation. The time has come to aggressively use proven nutrition and supplementation strategies to make your skin more beautiful, radiant, and resistant to the ravages of aging and wrinkling.

GAME PLAN FOR BETTER SKIN

By following the steps in this book, you can improve the health and appearance of your skin. It's not a complicated process. Here you will find a precise, no-nonsense game plan of nutrition and supplementation that is proven to help build and maintain beautiful, healthy skin for life. You'll also discover how to use this plan in conjunction with any other type of skin treatment or topical program that you currently follow. Specific nutrition and supplementation strategies are provided for use in combination with other standard treatments in the management of skin conditions such as acne; psoriasis; eczema; seborrhea; rosacea; dry, rough skin; and problems with poor complexion.

This resource explains in detail how you can incorporate nutrients into your skin-care program that are known to slow skin aging and help you to defend against skin damage induced by ultraviolet light, which leads to wrinkles, sunburn, and skin cancer. Documented cases illustrate how certain essential nutrients can reverse the appearance of fine lines and shallow wrinkles and help you understand how taking in these nutrients can help you preserve or recapture a more youthful appearance.

Supplementing your diet with precise levels of nutrients essential to skin health is the missing link to creating perfect looking skin. This book provides a step-by-step approach to transforming the science behind these findings into a program that leads to softer, smoother, healthier skin that looks and feels more elegant for life.

It may take many years before every skin-care professional fully understands these discoveries, but *The Wrinkle-Free Zone* gives you access to this cutting-edge information now. You can immediately begin your own skin-care management program in a safe, effective, and responsible fashion and soon reap the rewards of more beautiful skin. The most exciting news is that improvements in your skin's texture and appearance are detectable within thirty to sixty days of starting the Wrinkle-Free Zone Program—regardless of the quality of your skin when you begin.

In the following chapters, you're going to learn about the structure of the skin and how nutrients feed the young skin cells to make them strong. You're going to discover which supplements are most suitable for you and your conditions and concerns. Most important, you will be empowered to take charge of your skin care and gain the knowledge and direction needed to achieve optimal skin health.

It has been both a passion and a pleasure for me to have worked with patients over the past twenty years while researching and learning so much about this topic. I have seen the program detailed in this book help a great many people—patients, clients, family, and friends—to improve their complexion; reverse skin aging; reduce fine lines, wrinkles, and crow's feet; significantly reverse eczema, psoriasis, acne, and other skin conditions; and enjoy the softest, smoothest skin texture possible. The best part is that the program is easy to follow and incorporates only natural, safe nutrition and supplementation.

The most consistent finding in my work has been how pleased everyone is once they have experienced improvements in skin tone, texture, and appearance. I can't tell you how gratifying it has been for me to help people look and feel more attractive by showing them how to transform their skin into the soft, smooth, and radiant tissue that Nature intended it to be. I have also had the good fortune to travel across North America and teach the natural and effective strategies outlined here to thousands of estheticians, doctors, and other skin-care professionals at major conferences and conventions, and to publish my research in various professional publications. I hope you will find the subject fascinating and the program appealing. I'm confident you will be thrilled to discover how logical, convenient, and uncomplicated it is to have what you've always dreamed of: beautiful skin for life.

CHAPTER 1

Soft, Silky Skin for Life: The Role of Essential Oils

What's one of the best-kept secrets in the health and beauty world? It's really simple: By taking nutritional supplements, which include the right dosages and combinations of vitamins, minerals and essential oils, you can enhance the softness and smoothness of your skin, soften fine lines and wrinkles, and create a more beautiful and radiant complexion. Now, who doesn't want that? The basic nutritional program outlined in this chapter has been shown to do just that and has been proven effective in the treatment of eczema and an important component in the treatment of psoriasis.

However, before we discuss how nutritional supplements can improve skin quality, you need to know a few basics about how your skin develops and functions.

MEET YOUR SKIN

Over the many centuries of human existence, skin has not been treated very well. It's kind of like the Rodney Dangerfield of your body—it doesn't get enough respect. But as our scientific knowledge of this wondrous protective covering grows, we are beginning to understand more and more about how it works and what it needs to stay strong and healthy.

Skin Has Three Layers

Your skin is made up of three layers. The outer or surface layer is called the *epidermis,* a term with which you may be familiar. Next is the *dermis,* the layer that lies directly below the epidermis. Finally, we have the third layer called the *subcutis,* which is commonly referred to as the fat layer. Here's some basic information about these three layers and the unique function each performs in your overall health.

Epidermis

Despite being only as thick as a sheet of tissue paper, the epidermis is much hardier than you can imagine. This outer layer is comprised of tough keratin cells. These cells owe their strength to the fact that they're loaded with protein, the substance that gives them the toughness they need for their work on the surface. The epidermis also contains cells called melanocytes. These cells produce melanin, which determines the color of your skin.

By the time the keratin cells have developed in the bottom layer of the epidermis and worked their way to the top, they're dead. The protein that gives them their great strength is also the substance that kills them. As they emerge through the layers of the epidermis, they're worn away and replaced by new cells. These new skin cells are continually produced by basal cells, located at the bottom of the epidermis. Epidermal cells developing below the surface require optimal nutritional support to develop into healthy cells upon their arrival at the skin's surface, making the skin appear soft, moist, and beautiful.

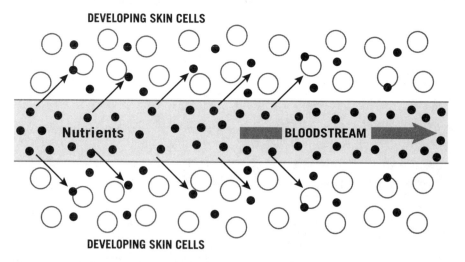

FIGURE 1.1. As nutrients flow through the bloodstream, they begin to nourish the developing skin cells in the skin's lower layers.

Dermis

The dermis is a resilient and elastic tissue that lies directly beneath the epidermis and makes up as much as 90 percent of the thickness of your skin. This is the layer where most of the skin's important functions take place. Among other things, the dermis contains hair follicles, blood vessels, sweat glands, and the nerves that help us sense temperature, pressure, and pain. Also found within the dermis are sweat glands that produce perspiration and sebaceous (oil) glands that secrete a thin coating of protective oil to act as a barrier and help protect against infections. Finally, the dermis contains elastin and collagen, two types of protein that help give your skin its elasticity and strength. Skin develops wrinkles when the collagen and elastin fibers in the dermis crosslink with each other in response to harmful molecules called free radicals, which are generated in the skin by overexposure to sunlight and environmental toxins. Fortunately, antioxidant nutrients, taken orally, can bolster your defenses against these free radicals and help prevent elastin and collagen crosslinks and, therefore, fine lines and wrinkles.

Subcutis

Found under the epidermis and dermis, the subcutis is composed mostly of fat, so it's known as the fat layer. It serves as a protector—think of it as a shock absorber—for the bones, muscles, and organs. The subcutis also acts as an insulator from the cold and as a storehouse of energy, and helps keep the skin looking smooth and plump.

Skin Facts

The skin is truly a remarkable work of nature. It's the body's largest organ, covering between 15 and 20 square feet. Measuring only one-twentieth of an inch thick, it can weigh as much as 20 pounds, also making it the body's heaviest organ. In every square inch of skin, you'll find many feet of blood vessels; dozens and dozens of oil glands; a couple hundred sensors for heat, cold, and pressure; 500 sweat glands; and more than 1,000 nerve endings.

This multilayered system constantly renews itself, shedding its dead top layer nonstop, every second of every day, while new cells formed in the deeper layers push to the surface. New cells are made at the same rate old cells die off and are rubbed, flaked, or washed off the top layer. Surface skin cells are completely replaced through this cycle approximately every twenty-seven days. The replacement of all the cells in the epidermal layers takes forty-five to seventy-four days on average.

Skin Serves Valuable Functions

What does your skin do? Let's imagine for a minute that your body is a fortress. Your skin is the outside wall, the first line of security in defense against the harsh outside forces that lead to disease and illness. Healthy skin can repel all sorts of attacks before they get a chance to take hold and work their way into your system. It effectively helps to protect you from outside elements, dangerous microbes, and other foreign substances.

The skin also helps to regulate your body temperature by releasing moisture in the form of sweat when your body begins to overheat. In the same manner, it aids in the body's detoxifying process, purging your system of many unwanted toxins through a complex "exhaust system." And skin gives you important temperature readings—for instance, if the sidewalk is too hot to walk on, or the water in the pool is too cold to jump into.

In many ways, skin is also your calling card. People tend to look first at someone's face when meeting them. Because your skin reflects your general health, a glowing complexion gives people you meet a positive impression of you as a person and of the lifestyle you lead. Of course, this works the other way, too. The skin reflects when we're seriously fatigued, ill, not eating properly, or when we're under some type of physical or emotional stress or strain. Skin doesn't lie. That's why the focus of *The Wrinkle-Free Zone* is on inner health and outer beauty; the two are inseparable. You can rest assured that as your body becomes healthier on the inside, your skin will become more beautiful on the outside when you implement the no-nonsense strategies of the Wrinkle-Free Zone Program.

Skin Differences between Women and Men

When it comes to achieving and maintaining healthy skin, the sad truth is that it's a lot more work for women than it is for men. One of the reasons for this is that women have thinner skin than men. That's because testosterone, the dominant hormone in men, causes male skin to be thicker, plumper, and fuller. To compound the situation, women's oil glands secrete slightly less oil than those of men. Therefore, women are more likely to experience dry skin.

As we grow older our hormone levels begin to change, resulting in thinner, more fragile skin for people of both sexes. In late middle age, men are affected when they begin to produce less testosterone, causing their skin to lose fullness. In women, however, the drop in hormone activity is more dramatic, and it has a greater effect. When women enter menopause, they experience a 90 percent drop in estrogen levels and a 66 percent drop in proges-terone levels, causing their skin to become dry and thin. Oil glands slow their production of natural emollients that keep the skin soft. As a result, the skin becomes a less efficient barrier against irritants, allergens, and bacteria mak-ing it more vulnerable to trauma and infections and more susceptible to a type of inflammation called dermatitis.

MAKING SKIN HEALTHY

Much can be done to make the skin not only look healthy but also function more efficiently in harmony with the body's other systems. When all your body's systems are getting the nourishment they need and are working together at peak efficiency, your health is better, you have more energy, and your skin is soft and smooth and has a healthy glow. All in all, you look better. It's the type of look you want, and your friends and family will notice. That is the promise of the Wrinkle-Free Zone Program.

Now that you understand the skin's structure and function, it's time to learn about the steps you need to take to make your skin look and feel great.

Your Skin Needs Good Fats

Yes, there is such a thing as good fats! And the bottom line is that everyone who supplements their diet with the right combination of these fats notices a marked improvement in their skin texture and appearance within the first month. It happens so fast because all the layers of the epidermis—not just the surface cells—are replaced by new cells every forty-five to seventy-four days. (As you might expect, younger people have faster turnover rates than older people.) So some very impressive changes occur within the first thirty days of supplementation, and by the end of two and a half to three months, most individuals report dramatic improvement in their skin's texture and appearance.

I also know from experience that many patients (and some doctors) are reluctant to believe that supplementation with vitamins, minerals, and essen-tial fats (fats that are necessary for normal cell structure and body functions but that our bodies cannot synthesize) can affect skin texture and appear-ance so dramatically. The very idea seems foreign to many people, so they begin the program with extreme skepticism. That may be the case because we've all been told that treating the topical layer of the skin is the only way to affect skin texture and appearance. We have been led to believe that cleansing, moisturizing, and applying topical lotions and treatments to the skin are the most important things we can do to improve skin health. But the truth is no matter how good a moisturizing cream you use, you can never achieve the level of soft, smooth skin that you have the potential to attain unless you provide your body with optimal dosages of essential fats and specific vitamins and minerals through nutritional supplementation. Take it from me, developing a healthy complexion and establishing permanent improvement in skin texture and appearance, as well as the resolution of some troublesome skin conditions, begins with the proper nourishment of skin cells from the inside-out.

In recent years, researchers have been able to determine the reason why the good fats (or fatty acids) found in borage, flaxseed, and fish oils are so critical to the maintenance of soft, smooth skin texture and the management of certain skin conditions. How do these fatty acids work? Investigative studies have shown the link between healthy skin texture and the intake of essential oils is the positive effect these unsaturated fats have on the development of prostaglandin (PG) hormones, which are synthesized within the epidermal skin cells. Studies show that the developing skin cells extract essential oils from the bloodstream and convert them into PG hormones. Once taken up by skin cells, the essential fats become one of three types of prostaglandin hormones: PG-1, PG-2, and PG-3.

While two of the three PG hormones are helpful for good skin, the other is destructive. The bad hormone is the one in the middle, PG-2. It makes the skin dry, rough, scaly, or flaky, whereas PG-1 and PG-3 make the skin soft, smooth, and moist. Unfortunately, the standard North American diet is loaded with the type of unsaturated fat that favors the production of PG-2. As a result, most people do not reach their potential for skin softness and smoothness, even if they are born with good genetics for skin texture.

Your Skin Does Not Need PG-2, the Bad Prostaglandin

Within the epidermal cells, PG-2 is formed from the unsaturated fat known as arachidonic acid (AA). You can bet that anything that rhymes with "demonic" and ends in "acid" is going to cause problems. AA is one of the bad fats concentrated in high-fat meats and dairy products. The more of these foods you eat, the greater the likelihood that PG-2 is the predominant prostaglandin hormone within your skin cells.

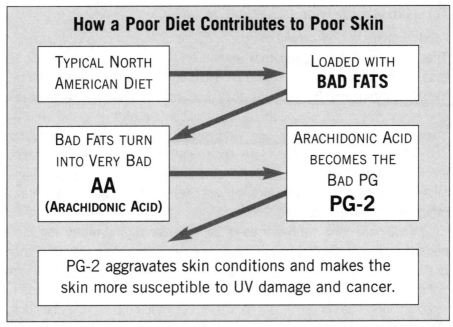

FIGURE 1.2. The typical North American diet encourages the development of the bad prostaglandin PG-2, which contributes to skin conditions and may lead to cancer.

If your skin is rough, dry, scaly, or flaky, your skin cells are most likely manufacturing more PG-2 than PG-1 and PG-3. In some people, symptoms appear, such as clusters of little dry, bumpy lesions, usually on the back, lower legs, buttocks, thighs, and backs and sides of the arms. This condition, known as perifollicular hyperkeratosis, is actually very common, though many health practitioners are not familiar with scientific studies showing that it is most often caused by an essential fatty acid deficiency (vitamin A deficiency may also be present). It can be completely cured by supplementation with a combination of borage, flaxseed, and fish oils.

The overabundance of AA and other unsaturated fats in the standard North American diet also contributes to a host of complexion problems and aggravates skin conditions like eczema and psoriasis. Experimental studies show that skin cells with a high concentration of AA are more prone to inflammatory problems and even cancerous changes upon exposure to ultraviolet light. The conversion of AA to PG-2 produces an effect where skin cells divide at a much faster rate, making them more likely to exhibit inflammatory responses and cancerous mutations.

Foods to Avoid, Foods That Are Healthy

Foods that are loaded with AA are best avoided or at least eaten infrequently. That's different from saying they should be "consumed in moderation." Indeed, the following foods should be avoided as much as possible: all red meats, including hamburgers and steak; pork products such as bacon, ham, and spare ribs; most cold cuts, with the exception of turkey and chicken breast; organ meats; and egg yolks. Additionally, you should avoid dairy products with a high concentration of AA, especially butter, cream, cream cheese, whole milk (homogenized), and any cheese that is higher than 3 percent milk fat—which includes most of them—as well as any milk or yogurt that contains more than 1-percent milk fat.

In addition, corn, sunflower seed, safflower seed, and mixed vegetable oils should be banned from your diet and never again appear in your kitchen or pantry shelves. *Ever.* Why the hard line with these oils? Simply put, they're not good for you or your skin because they are a rich source of an unsaturated fat known as linoleic acid (LA). It's important to note that the body does require small amounts of LA in the range of about 1 percent of our total daily calories. If you can stay close to that number, you're fine. But in North America we're fighting a losing battle, as the average person eats a daily diet that contains between 7 and 10 percent LA out of the total calories consumed. This overwhelms the body with LA, and when the body has used all it needs, the rest is converted into AA—which, in turn, is converted by skin cells to PG-2. That's why corn, sunflower seed, safflower seed, and mixed vegetable oils should be viewed as indirect sources of AA and avoided whenever possible.

What vegetable oils are healthy? Olive, canola, and peanut oils each provide about all the body really needs of LA. These oils are also richly endowed with a monounsaturated fat known as oleic acid, which is associated with reduced risk of heart disease and some cancers. Unlike AA, the monounsaturated fat found in olive, canola, and peanut oils does not get converted into prostaglandin hormones by the body, and thus does not contribute to the formation of PG-2 within skin cells.

By now you've probably realized that you're going to have to make some adjustments—major or minor—to your diet. Chicken, turkey, fish, and soy products are better sources of protein. Choose 1-percent or nonfat milk and yogurt, and avoid cheeses that are above 3-percent milk fat content, as well as butter, sour cream, and the like. By cutting down on these foods, you will not only improve the quality of your skin by reducing the synthesis of PG-2,

---

Oil Hit List

To avoid the disastrous effects of PG-2, it's crucial to avoid the oils on this hit list:

- CORN OIL
- SAFFLOWER SEED OIL
- SUNFLOWER SEED OIL
- MIXED VEGETABLE OIL

Why? These oils are loaded with linoleic acid, which the body converts to PG-2.

---

but you'll also reduce your risk of heart attack, stroke, and some cancers, especially colon and reproductive organ cancers. This is because the animal foods that are loaded with AA are also the same animal foods that are loaded with saturated fat, which is known to drive up blood cholesterol levels, increase cancer risk, and promote weight gain and obesity. So you are doing yourself a huge favor by restricting your intake of the foods listed above.

However, if changing your diet seems too drastic at this point, don't despair. Even if you only follow the supplementation program outlined at the end of this chapter, you will still see significant improvement in the softness and smoothness of your skin within the first month, with even greater changes by the end of the third month. So don't panic about making all the suggested dietary changes overnight. Start by taking the recommended supplements and slowly make adjustments to your diet over time to lower your intake of AA and saturated fat. The most important point is that all the measures to reduce the synthesis of PG-2 discussed in this chapter should be taken seriously sooner rather than later.

The Good Oils

No need to cut all the oils out of your diet. Here's a list of the healthy oils:

- OLIVE OIL
- CANOLA OIL
- PEANUT OIL

These oils contain levels of LA that are ideally suited to your body's needs.

The Good News about PG-1

The key building block for the "good" PG-1 is an unsaturated fat known as GLA (gamma-linolenic acid), which is found in high concentrations in borage oil. In North America, we all have suboptimal levels of GLA in our bodies. Without supplementation, it's difficult for skin cells to get sufficient amounts of GLA to create the levels of PG-1 necessary to make the skin as smooth and soft as possible. This is because there are no good food sources of GLA, and although GLA can be formed in the body from LA, the body can't make the optimal levels necessary to maximize skin softness and smoothness. In fact, many individuals have trouble making GLA from LA due to a defect in an enzyme known as delta-6 desaturase, which is necessary for this conversion. For instance, individuals with diabetes, PMS, and eczema have been shown to have this defect. The consumption of alcohol, refined sugars, and hydrogenated fats also tends to inhibit the conversion of LA to GLA. Even the aging process itself slows the conversion of LA to GLA, as the enzyme becomes more sluggish over the years.

Everyone Needs Supplementation with Borage Oil

Clinical evidence demonstrates that everyone benefits from GLA supplementation with borage oil. It improves skin texture even in people who have reasonably soft skin to begin with and makes a dramatic change in people whose skin is dry, rough, or scaly. GLA supplementation has also been used successfully in the treatment of eczema and other skin conditions. I recommend that patients get their GLA supplementation from borage oil, as it is the most cost-effective source. But that alone is not enough to give you the skin you deserve. The trick is to take borage oil in a combination supplement that also contains the omega-3 fats found in flaxseed oil and a fish oil (30 percent EPA and 20 percent DHA). These omega-3 fats work together with borage oil to produce absolutely beautiful, luscious skin that is smooth, soft, silky, and radiant.

Supplementing with omega-3 fats from flaxseed and fish oils also inhibits the conversion of LA to AA by blocking delta-5 desaturase, the enzyme needed to convert LA into AA. This means less buildup of PG-2 within your skin cells.

Vitamins and Minerals Are Also Needed to Make PG-1

It's important to understand that the conversion of GLA to PG-1 within epidermal cells also requires adequate amounts of certain vitamins and minerals,

---

Success Story
Master CM Conquers Childhood Eczema

MASTER CM WAS A FIVE-YEAR-OLD BOY who suffered from childhood eczema, or atopic dermatitis. His mother attended one of my nutrition seminars and was curious to see if any kind of dietary change or supplement program could help her son conquer this troublesome problem. She mentioned that the doctor and specialist they had seen recommended the use of a topical cortisone cream, but the cream was causing his skin to become very thin and did not satisfactorily resolve the problem. I explained that many cases of childhood eczema were caused by the body's inability to make adequate amounts of PG-1 for skin health due to a genetic defect in the enzyme that converts the essential fatty acid LA into GLA. I suggested we place her son on a clinical trial using an essential oils supplement, which included GLA and other essential fatty acids, as well as the vitamins and minerals necessary to convert the essential oils into PG-1 and PG-3. (I adjusted the dosages to suit the child's body.)

Within one month, Master CM showed me that the eczema lesions once all over his body had completely cleared up. In the months that followed, none of the lesions returned, and his mother told me proudly many months later that the supplementation program had cured her son. When she reported to the doctor and specialist that her son's case had been cured by the right combination and dosages of nutritional supplements, they had listened to her in disbelief. But they couldn't refute the facts.

---

including vitamin B_6, zinc, and magnesium. These vitamins and minerals act as helpers or cofactors in the enzyme reactions that convert GLA to PG-1; if they are not available in sufficient amounts, the conversion of GLA to PG-1 does not occur at a normal pace and may even be completely inhibited. Thus, there is a marriage between the intake of essential oils and the need to supplement your diet with the vitamins and minerals powering the enzyme reactions that convert GLA into PG-1. The amounts of the various vitamins and minerals required to convert essential fats into PG-1 and PG-3 are summarized at the end of this chapter.

Why PG-3 Is Good for You

The very versatile PG-3 serves many purposes. It is known to reduce inflammation, including skin inflammatory responses—a role it shares with PG-1. In fact, PG-1 and PG-3 work together to create skin that is smooth, soft, silky, and moist. PG-3 is formed from the omega-3 unsaturated fat known as eicosapentaenoic acid (EPA), which is found in cold-water marine life—salmon, mackerel, anchovies, sardines, and tuna—and in fish oil supplements that contain EPA. The body can also convert the omega-3 fat known as alpha-linolenic acid (ALA) into EPA, thereby increasing the production of PG-3. ALA is found in rich concentrations in flaxseed oil with an approximately 58 percent yield. In fact, flaxseed oil is the world's most abundant source of ALA, and for this reason, it is a very desirable nutritional supplement for skin health and appearance.

Taking dietary supplements that contain flaxseed oil and a high-yield fish oil has been shown to significantly increase the body's production of PG-3, resulting in improved skin texture and appearance and helping to combat cer-

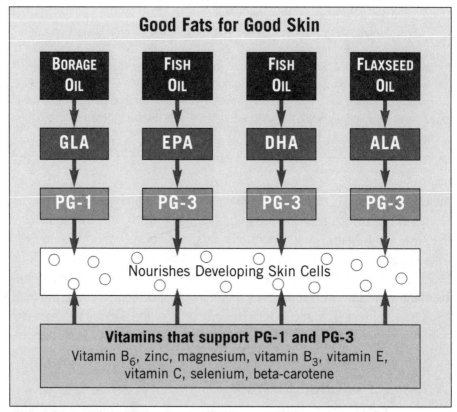

FIGURE 1.3. Everyone needs some fat in their diet. Flax, borage, and fish oils support healthy skin.

tain skin conditions like psoriasis and eczema. Fish oil also contains another unsaturated fat called docosahexaenoic acid (DHA), which the body can convert into EPA and PG-3, if required. As a bonus, DHA also promotes the development and function of the brain and is important for good vision.

PG-3 for Total Body Wellness

In addition to improving the softness and smoothness of your skin, PG-3 is very important for total body wellness, as it reduces the risk of heart attacks by dilating, or widening, blood vessels and lessens abnormal blood clotting. PG-3 has also been shown to reduce cancer risk by slowing cell division rates. Typically, the body's natural DNA repair enzymes can keep up with normal cell division rates and correct any genetic mistakes. But when cells divide at an accelerated rate, enzymes can't keep up with the repairs. The result is increased genetic mutations and increased formation of cancer cells.

In particular, PG-3 may be effective in the prevention of skin cancer. Research shows omega-3 fats slowed the division rate of skin cells by promoting the formation of PG-3, which helps reduce the incidence of mutations and inflammatory conditions, even when cells are exposed to ultraviolet light. Thus, omega-3 fat supplementation may help guard against the development of skin cancer, in addition to slowing skin aging. In contrast, experimental studies have shown that higher PG-2 levels in skin cells promoted significantly more cancer development when cells were exposed to ultraviolet light than did skin cells with lower concentrations of PG-2.

There is also evidence that PG-3 levels may be linked to the risk of breast cancer. Some studies show, for instance, that women with higher levels of ALA in the fat cells within their breast tissue have a lower subsequent risk of developing breast cancer than women with lower ALA concentrations. Researchers believe that the conversion of ALA to PG-3 helps to protect breast cells from undergoing malignant changes.

Many researchers studying the role of essential fats in the human diet suggest that most North Americans have an imbalance in the ratio of omega-3 to omega-6 fats. For the most part, we ingest too many foods rich in AA and LA and too little omega-3 fats. In turn, this contributes to an increased risk of heart disease, stroke, certain cancers, inflammatory states, and other problems because of an overproduction of PG-2 in body tissues.

The bottom line is that we all need to increase our omega-3 fat intake, and when we do, our skin looks and feels better—and we get a whole bunch

Success Story
Miss J and Her Parents Enhance Their Skin

WHEN SHE CAME TO MY OFFICE, Miss J was a forty-year-old woman who had suffered from a serious kidney affliction and had only one functional kidney. Aware that the kidneys are an important organ of elimination, she had developed a keen interest in nutrition and supplementation over the years in an attempt to prevent any damage to her one healthy kidney and to optimize her health as much as possible. She was already taking a multitude of nutritional supplements when she consulted with me about nutrition and lifestyle. Aware that certain supplements could play a role in skin health and appearance, Miss J also expressed interest in a supplement or topical lotion that might improve her complexion and skin texture. In truth, she had taken good care of her skin over the years and had no significant skin or complexion problems. I introduced her to the essential oils supplement and the high-potency multivitamin and mineral supplement (to be discussed in Chapter 2) and explained that the ingredients were more complete and better balanced than what she had been using.

Within two to four weeks of switching supplements, she found her skin was smoother, softer, and moister than she had ever experienced and that many of the fine lines on her face had softened or completely disappeared. She was so excited about the changes that she told her parents, and her father immediately requested the supplements. Within a few weeks, he reported that his skin was much improved, the lines on his face were reduced (he claims some disappeared), and he was looking and feeling much younger. His wife, who was at first quite skeptical, thought at first that her daughter and husband were imagining things, but eventually she couldn't help noticing how much younger, radiant, and less wrinkled her husband's face had become, and that his skin was noticeably softer and smoother. So Miss J's mother insisted on getting her own batch of supplements so she, too, could join the family anti-aging movement.

Miss J was amazed that the essential oils supplement and less-potent multivitamin she had been taking didn't give her the kind of skin benefits the new formulas provided. I explained that her original essential oils supplement was missing GLA, from which skin cells make PG-1, and that the absence of just one important ingredient like that, or an insufficient amount of one or more ingredients, can prevent the skin from being as beautiful and elegant as possible.

of other health benefits, too. The best thing you can do now to improve your skin is to take an essential oils supplement that contains borage, flaxseed, and fish oils at the recommended dosages.

Vitamins and Minerals Are Needed for Prostaglandin Synthesis

I can't stress enough that your body needs the help of certain vitamins and minerals to convert the essential fats in borage, flaxseed, and fish oils into PG-1 and PG-3. Taking in suboptimal amounts of these nutrients is like putting high-octane gas into your car but then disconnecting the battery. Even a full tank of that high-octane fuel will be of no benefit until you reconnect the battery and start the engine because all systems must be operating and working in unison for the car to run properly. In much the same way, you must take the vitamins and minerals required for the enzymatic reactions that enable skin cells to convert essential oils into PG-1 and PG-3 to achieve healthy, radiant skin.

For example, the efficient conversion of ALA to EPA requires sufficient amounts of vitamin B_6, niacin (vitamin B_3), zinc, and magnesium. The synthesis of PG-1 and PG-3 also requires recommended daily dosages of vitamin C, vitamin E, and selenium. These nutrients act as antioxidants, which destroy harmful elements in the body and help slow skin aging and wrinkling. They also affect the action of cyclooxygenase, the final enzyme needed in the conversion of GLA and EPA to PG-1 and PG-3, respectively.

STEP-BY-STEP NUTRITIONAL AND SUPPLEMENTATION PROGRAM

Clinical and investigative studies now confirm that supplementation with a combination of flaxseed, borage, and fish oils at the correct dosages creates softer, smoother skin in virtually every individual who takes the dosages recommended in this chapter. This program also helps to improve complexion and soften fine lines and wrinkles and can be an important component in the treatment of skin disorders such as eczema, psoriasis, perifollicular hyperkeratosis, and acne. This is due to the effects of GLA, ALA, and EPA in promoting the synthesis of PG-1 and PG-3 within developing skin cells. Emerging experimental data show that higher concentrations of omega-3 fats in skin cells may offer additional protection against ultraviolet light-induced skin cancer, as well as skin aging caused by sunlight (known as photo-aging) and wrinkling of the skin.

Success Story
Miss L Adopts the Wrinkle-Free Program

Miss L, a woman in her early forties, was concerned because she continued to experience small breakouts of acne, and her skin was often dry and was not as smooth as she desired. She took the essential oils supplement and the high-potency multivitamin and mineral supplement (discussed in Chapter 2) as a sixty-day clinical trial to see if she would notice any improvement. At the end of the two-month period, she was excited by how soft, smooth, and moist her skin had become, seemingly overnight. The breakouts of acne she had experienced stopped almost completely since she began the program, and she found she needed to use much less moisturizer than before.

"My face no longer feels tight and dry after I shower," she told me. "I feel like the skin on my face retains its moisture even while I shower, which is unusual for me. Normally, I feel like I have to put a ton of moisturizer on my face immediately after showering to prevent my face from tightening up from the dryness."

The calluses on the sides of her fingers from frequent summer gardening had also softened significantly, although she continued to use gardening tools as much as ever. Her skin no longer bruised as easily as it once had, and small cuts that she frequently experienced healed much faster than they had before she started taking the recommended supplements. Prior to starting the program, she considered herself to be a bit of a "klutz" because she was always bruising or injuring herself, so she soon noticed the difference supplementation made. Extremely pleased with the results, Miss L has faithfully followed the Wrinkle-Free Zone Program since her first visit.

Essential fatty acid supplementation must be viewed as an important component of lifelong skin-care management for everyone. Recommended doses of certain vitamins and minerals are required to efficiently convert GLA found in borage oil to PG-1 and ALA, and EPA from flaxseed and fish oils, respectively, to PG-3.

That's the story of how your skin can become softer, smoother, silkier, and more radiant within the first thirty days of the program. Just follow the steps summarized below, and you'll be amazed at how quickly you will start to see real, lasting changes in your complexion. Here's a practical step-by-step daily formula:

1. To reduce the buildup of arachidonic acid and the resulting PG-2 syn-

thesis, avoid or restrict your intake of high-fat meat and dairy products. Chicken, turkey, soy products, and fish are good alternatives, as well as 1-percent or nonfat milk and yogurt, and cheeses that are less than 4 percent milk fat. Substitute olive, canola, and peanut oils for corn, sunflower seed, safflower seed, and mixed vegetable oils in salad dressings, and for making stir-fries and sautéing vegetables. Consume alcohol in moderation, if at all, and reduce your intake of refined sugars and hydrogenated fats.

2. To enhance the production of PG-1 and PG-3, which improve the softness and smoothness of the skin and help alleviate certain skin conditions, supplement your diet with an all-in-one essential fatty acid supplement. I formulated a supplement that provides 400 milligrams (mg) each of flaxseed, borage, and fish oils in a 1,200 mg capsule for my patients and for use by other skin-care professionals. For best results, take two to three capsules daily. (Individuals with very dry skin, eczema, or psoriasis may require up to six capsules a day to reverse these conditions.) The fish oils should yield 30 percent EPA and 20 percent DHA content, and the borage and flaxseed oils should be from GMO-free sources, meaning that they do not come from genetically modified seeds. I would also encourage you to eat lots of fish and soy products.

3. To facilitate the conversion of essential fats to PG-1 and PG-3, you should take a high-potency multivitamin and mineral formula that provides the following daily dosages: 1,000 mg vitamin C, 400 international units (IU) of all-natural vitamin E, 10,000 IU beta-carotene, 100 micrograms (mcg) selenium, 15 mg zinc, 2,500 IU vitamin A, and a vitamin B-50 complex, as well as other vitamins and minerals that support skin health and appearance, which we will discuss in Chapter 2.

Essential fatty acid supplementation, in conjunction with optimal intakes of key vitamins and minerals, have been the missing link in skin-care management for many years. From clinical experience, I can assure you that you'll notice a positive improvement in skin texture and smoothness, most likely within the first month of following this program. (See Resources.) Scientific studies and clinical experience confirm that by following the simple recommendations outlined in this book, you will experience softer, smoother, more radiant skin within the first thirty days.

Keep in mind, however, that this is a lifelong strategy, as all the skin cells within the epidermis are replaced by new cells every forty-five to seventy-four days. Because developing skin cells require a constant daily supply of essential nutrients, that means you must faithfully follow this dietary and supplementation program seven days a week, 365 days a year, and you won't be disappointed. That alone should motivate you to follow the Wrinkle-Free Zone Program consistently for the rest of your life.

CHAPTER 2

Slowing Skin Aging
and Preventing Wrinkles:
The Role of Nutritional
Antioxidants

I n Chapter 1 you learned about the importance of supplementation with essential oils. This chapter will teach you about the essential nutrients that help slow the aging process of your skin, prevent wrinkles, and reduce your risk of skin cancer.

The story begins when we look at the damage that sunlight wreaks on the skin. For a long time we have been told that ultraviolet (UV) light from the sun and tanning beds can damage the skin, accelerate skin aging and wrinkling, and increase skin cancer risk. This happens because some UV light actually penetrates through the skin and scatters through all the layers of the epidermis and the dermis. The UV light doesn't hurt the surface skin cells because they're dead. But that isn't the case for the cells below the surface. Subsurface skin cells are alive, and they need oxygen to help power their biological machinery. When UV light enters these living skin cells, it converts some of the oxygen in the cells into oxygen-free radicals, commonly referred to as free radicals.

OXYGEN-FREE RADICALS: THE ENEMY WITHIN

The term "free radical" sounds like something from the hippie movement in the 1960s. If only they were as harmless and nonthreatening as that! The truth is that free radicals can cause immense harm in your body, including serious damage to your skin.

Here's how it happens in very simple terms. The oxygen contained in your skin cells is a very volatile substance. It can easily pick up some of the electron energy that incoming UV light brings to the body. The problems start

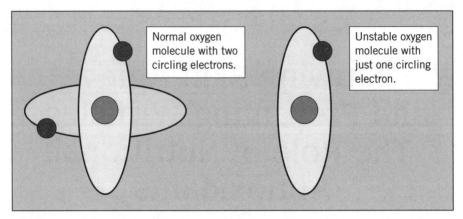

Normal oxygen molecule with two circling electrons.

Unstable oxygen molecule with just one circling electron.

FIGURE 2.1. Free radicals create havoc when they roam the body, stealing electrons to stabilize themselves.

when an oxygen molecule becomes activated by picking up only one electron from the UV light. At that point, the molecule becomes very unstable and aggressive. Why? Electrons circle the nucleus of an atom in pairs, and this pairing ensures balance and stability. When only one electron is added to the oxygen molecule, this balance is lost, and the nature of the molecule changes. Simply put, it goes from a calm, law-abiding citizen to Attila the Hun—it has become a free radical. The oxygen-free radical desperately begins to scavenge around within the skin cell for an electron it can steal from another molecule in order to complete the pair and return to stability. Once the oxygen free radical steals the electron it needs from a neighboring molecule, the oxygen molecule becomes stable once more.

However, this creates a whole new problem, as the neighboring molecule, which was minding its own business, loses an electron. Having been robbed of an electron, this molecule now begins a frantic search to find another electron to restabilize itself. This sets off a domino effect, with free radicals robbing other molecules of electrons, which in turn creates more free radicals, and so forth. The only way to stop this progression is to add an antioxidant nutrient or enzyme into the mix. The antioxidant quenches or neutralizes the free-radical chain reaction.

One way to picture this scenario is if you envision that the newly formed oxygen-free radical is the leader of a street gang who goes door-to-door recruiting other kids to join his gang. Pretty soon, they have formed their own little army, and then they're off, smashing windows, kicking in doors, and

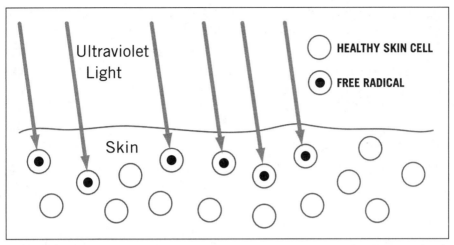

FIGURE 2.2. When UV light hits the skin, it penetrates all layers. In the process, it injects healthy skin cells with a single electron, turning them into damaging free radicals. As they roam the cells in search of a second electron to pair with, the free radicals steal electrons from other cellular components, creating more free-radical damage in the process.

dumping garbage cans all over the street. Those kids can do a lot of damage to a community. Likewise, the oxygen-free radicals created from UV light exposure can do a great deal of permanent damage to your skin cells.

Cigarette smoking causes lung cancer in the same way that UV light affects skin cells. Free radicals contained in cigarette smoke cause damage to the DNA material within lung cells. If enough damage is inflicted, then a mutation occurs in the DNA template and allows cancerous changes to occur in a once healthy lung cell.

Oxygen-free radicals created by UV light exposure have been shown to damage the proteins in our skin cells, as well as the genetic material contained in DNA; the outer skin of the cell, known as the cell membrane; and many other cellular elements.

When this occurs, the skin undergoes more rapid aging, known as photoaging. Proteins within the dermal layer become crosslinked, causing wrinkles to appear, and DNA damage to skin cells begins to accumulate, increasing the risk of cancerous mutations and setting the stage for skin cancer to develop. Free-radical damage from UV light exposure creates mutations that are known to lead to the development of skin cancer—basal cell carcinoma, squamous cell carcinoma, and melanoma. Currently, nonmelanoma skin cancer is the most common malignancy in the United States, and the estimated lifetime risk of developing malignant melanoma for Americans has risen from 1 in 250 in 1981 to 1 in 87 in 1996. Likewise, aging spots seem to result from a similar process, as skin cells become filled with a debris known as lipofuscin pigment from extensive free-radical damage to various cellular components.

Cumulative lifetime sun exposure and decreased protection from the earth's thinning ozone layer are the primary culprits for these disquieting statistics. Too much sun exposure leads to sunburn, which is an inflammation of the skin caused in part by sunlight's activation of free radical molecules. Excessive sun exposure also impairs the skin's genetic material contained in DNA and RNA, as well as reduces immune function, which further increases the risk of skin cancer. No matter how careful you are about exposing your skin to the sun, some ultraviolet light waves will penetrate through your suntan lotion's protective antioxidant shield and generate free radicals within your skin cells, and those cells need all the help they can get to resist wrinkling and related skin damage.

The Link between Pheomelanin and Skin Cancer

People with fair skin and red hair, who have red-brown or yellow freckles or skin pigment, are at higher risk for developing skin cancer from free radicals generated by UV light than are individuals with freckles and skin pigment that is brown or black. That is because these two types of melanin pigments are very different in structure and function.

Cells called melanocytes, which are interspersed throughout epidermal and dermal skin layers, synthesize melanin pigment and literally inject it into neighboring skin cells—especially the epidermal cells. Melanin pigment formation is greatly increased when the skin is exposed to UV light from the sun or from tanning beds, and this increased synthesis and injection of these pigments into epidermal cells gives the skin its tanned appearance after exposure to UV light exposure. This is the case in individuals who produce brown or black melanin pigment, known as eumelanin, due to their genetic structure. Eumelanin is actually an antioxidant that acts as a shield within the skin, absorbing photo energy from UV light and thereby helping to reduce free-radical damage. Increased eumelanin production and distribution throughout the skin is the body's natural response when it senses increased bombardment from free radicals induced by UV light. Eumelanin helps reduce the potential for future free-radical damage that the skin cells sense is imminent. But before the tan appears, substantial free-radical damage has probably already occurred, because the skin has come under attack from free radicals. The tan is an attempt to minimize the damage should you again be exposed to UV light in the near future. That is why dermatologists warn that there is no such thing as a "healthy" tan.

However, if you are exposed to sunlight or use a tanning bed on occasion—as many people do—it is far better to make eumelanin than melanin that is red-brown or yellow because that type of melanin, known as pheomelanin, is very dangerous. Rather than acting as a shield when the skin is exposed to UV light, it instead enhances free-radical damage to the skin, and may even damage the DNA structure of the melanocyte cells themselves. This is what researchers believe leads to the development of melanoma, a highly lethal form of skin cancer that has escalated at an alarming rate in recent years.

It may be that fair-skinned, red-haired people who make pheomelanin upon exposure to sunlight would benefit from more antioxidant supplementation, as discussed below, than people whose cells produce eumelanin. In my view, everyone should fortify their nutritional antioxidant defenses with a healthy diet and supplementation, as skin cancer continues to affect more and more people every year, and not just those with red-brown or yellow skin pigment, who are typically at greater risk.

Smoking and Alcohol Also Create Free Radicals

Besides potentially harmful UV rays, there are other sources of free radicals that can damage skin cells in a similar fashion. Two main culprits are cigarette smoke and alcohol consumption. Cigarette smoke is loaded with many different free radical agents that can cause serious damage to tissues throughout the body, including skin cells. This is why 87 percent of those who develop lung cancer are cigarette smokers and why smokers are three times as likely as nonsmokers to develop premature wrinkles. Smoking is also associated with stomach, mouth, and esophageal cancers, among others. In fact, the National Cancer Institute has published research papers indicating that approximately 30 percent of all human cancers result from cigarette smoking.

Poor diets also account for 35 percent of all cancers. One significant factor is the overconsumption of alcohol, which is associated with approximately 3 percent of all cancers, according to research published in the

Journal of the National Cancer Institute. Alcohol consumption generates free radicals when it is broken down by the liver. Once formed, these free radicals roam around the body and cause damage to many different tissues. This is one of the reasons why the faces of people with alcoholism often have a characteristic appearance, showing signs of accelerated aging and premature wrinkling.

I strongly suggest that you don't smoke and that you limit your alcohol consumption to no more than one drink per day, as the body seems able to safely metabolize only one alcoholic drink within a twenty-four-hour period without increasing free-radical production. That point is best illustrated by the Health Professionals Follow-up Study and the Nurses Health Study both of which show that consistently drinking two or three alcoholic drinks a day is associated with a two- to three-times greater risk of developing colon and breast cancers.

ANTIOXIDANT SUPPLEMENTS TO THE RESCUE

Premature aging of the skin, including accelerated wrinkling and damage to the genetic material of epidermal and other skin cells—melanocytes, for example—is known to result from free-radical damage. That is why for many years now the medical profession and other leading health authorities have told us to avoid overexposure to sunlight and other known sources of free radicals, to wear protective clothing, and to use antioxidant-rich sunblock to minimize our risk of skin damage from ultraviolet light. These, of course, are all important measures to reduce the risk of skin cancer, as well as to prevent wrinkles and premature skin aging.

Recent evidence has shown that you should also be taking a multivitamin and mineral supplement each day that is enriched with antioxidant vitamins and minerals. Antioxidants are agents that intercept, quench, and neutralize free radicals and convert them into harmless substances that the body can eliminate. Scientific studies have demonstrated that antioxidant protection works from the inside-out, meaning that antioxidant vitamins and minerals are picked up from the bloodstream by developing epidermal cells below the skin's surface. The higher your antioxidant intake, the higher the antioxidant concentrations are within your skin cells, and the greater protection these free-radical quenchers afford.

Some of the premier nutritional antioxidants that protect the skin from the inside-out are vitamins C and E, beta-carotene, selenium, zinc, copper, mag-

Success Story
Miss CB Sees Many Improvements

MISS CB WAS A FIFTY-FIVE-YEAR-OLD WOMAN who was taking a number of heart medications that were known to cause skin dryness. After a serious health challenge several months before, Miss CB had noticed that the skin above her eyes had become quite puffy and wrinkled—to quote her, like "the earth after a small earthquake." I suggested she start nourishing her skin with the high-potency multivitamin and mineral supplement and the essential oils supplement.

A little over two months later, Miss CB was delighted that despite taking the heart medications, she could see a significant reduction in the wrinkles above her eyes; moreover, her skin had become extremely soft, moist, and radiant. Indeed, many of her friends and family had commented on how good her skin looked since she started the supplementation program. She also noted that she didn't need to use as much hand cream and moisturizer to keep her skin soft and smooth. She reported that her hair, which had begun thinning, had instead become thicker. When she tried stopping the program to see what would happen, she soon felt tired and less healthy, similar to how she had been feeling before starting supplementation. She also told me that during the summer months she would usually develop cracks along the sides of her heels from walking barefoot, but not when she was following the program.

As an interesting side note, Miss CB told me that professionally she formulates gourmet dog food, and having experienced success with the supplementation program herself, she now includes essential oils like GLA and EPA in her products. Not surprisingly, her clients rave about the sheen and luster of their dogs' coats.

nesium, and manganese. Antioxidant enzymes within skin cells include catalase, glutathione peroxidase, and superoxide dismutase. It seems the minerals selenium, zinc, copper, magnesium, and manganese boost your antioxidant defenses by activating antioxidant enzymes; thus, without adequate amounts of these minerals, antioxidant enzymes cannot effectively neutralize free radicals. The body's genetic code instructs each cell to make antioxidant enzymes, but they cannot perform their protective duties without the aid of important minerals. This illustrates how genetic factors depend upon optimal nutrition for the body to work properly.

Studies indicate that the level of antioxidants required to provide skin cells with maximum protection from UV light during the normal course of living is well above that which can be provided by diet alone. Even though it's certainly helpful to eat lots of fruits and vegetables, it seems that dietary intake alone is not enough antioxidant insurance to afford the skin with maximum protection against premature wrinkling, skin aging, and skin cancer over a lifetime. That's why I created a high-potency multivitamin and mineral formula to optimize UV protection and enhance skin health and appearance that includes the following: 1,000 milligrams (mg) vitamin C, 400 international units (IU) vitamin E (all natural), 10,000 IU beta-carotene, 2,500 IU vitamin A, 100 micrograms (mcg) selenium, 15 mg zinc, 50 mg bioflavonoids, 2 mg copper, 200 mg magnesium, and 5 mg manganese. The complete formula is outlined in the table you'll find at the end of this chapter.

Antioxidant Research and the Skin

Research indicates that antioxidant supplements are a crucial component in preventing skin wrinkling and possibly cancer development. A study by B. Eberlein-Konig and fellow researchers published in *The Journal of the American Academy of Dermatology* illustrates this point extremely well. In this double-blind, placebo-controlled study, human subjects were given either an antioxidant supplement or a placebo each day for a number of weeks. After several weeks of supplementation, subjects in both groups had areas of their skin exposed to a moderate to high dose of UV light for a specified length of time. The study demonstrated that subjects who were given vitamin C and E supplements showed significantly less free-radical damage to their skin after UV light exposure than did the group given the placebo. The group taking the antioxidant supplements also showed significantly less sunburn reaction. Other studies have shown that free radicals—especially those caused by sun exposure—deplete the skin of its antioxidant defenses quite rapidly, further increasing the need for antioxidant intake to replenish the depleted antioxidant supplies within the skin cells.

Vitamin C

Vitamin C is a water-soluble vitamin that serves many purposes in the body. It is required for production of the cartilage between your bones, as well as for collagen synthesis, which strengthens blood vessels, including those on the face, helping to prevent broken blood vessel patches. The vitamin also supports immune function and detoxification processes and is required for the synthesis of important brain chemicals. A powerful antioxidant extracted from the bloodstream by skin cells, vitamin C has been shown to help protect skin cells from free radicals generated by exposure to sunlight. Clinical and exper-imental studies also demonstrate that it's an important anti-aging vitamin that slows skin aging, reduces wrinkling, and helps prevent genetic damage to skin cells that has been associated with skin cancer.

The available data indicate that most people should supplement their diet with 500 to 2,000 mg vitamin C daily to help slow skin aging and wrinkling and to reduce general free-radical damage to the body. The secondary ben-efits of this level of vitamin C supplementation include a healthier immune system, stronger blood vessels with less leaking and vein varicosities, reduced risk of cataracts, and according to some studies, lower risk of stomach and colon cancers.

Vitamin E

Vitamin E is also a powerful antioxidant vitamin, but, unlike vitamin C, it is fat-soluble, not water-soluble. That means vitamin E can protect skin cells in places where vitamin C cannot—the outer fatty skin, or membrane, that sur-rounds each individual skin cell, and the membrane that surrounds the genet-ic material of the cell contained in the cell nucleus. Free-radical damage from UV light is known to cause extensive damage to both the skin's cell membrane and the nuclear membrane that, in turn, results in accelerated aging of the skin, the formation of aging spots, and genetic mutations to the skin's DNA. Supplementation with vitamin E has been shown to reduce these effects.

Studies suggest that 400 IU natural vitamin E taken as a daily supplement is a prudent dosage to help optimize protection of skin cells. This level of sup-plementation also helps skin cells make the prostaglandin hormones PG-1 and PG-3, which help make the skin softer and smoother. Additional health benefits of taking the recommended dose of vitamin E include protection against heart attacks; Alzheimer's disease; cataracts; and macular degenera-tion, which is the leading cause of blindness in people over age fifty-five.

Skin cells require both the water-soluble antioxidants in vitamin C and the fat-soluble antioxidants in vitamin E and beta-carotene at optimal doses to protect the many different cellular structures from free-radical damage. The two vitamins work with essential oil supplementation (as discussed in Chap-ter 1) and B vitamins (discussed below) to make the skin softer, smoother, and more radiant.

OTHER VITAMINS AND MINERALS FOR SKIN HEALTH AND APPEARANCE

By now I hope you're convinced that antioxidant supplements are a necessary part of an anti-aging, anti-wrinkle, and skin cancer prevention program and that it takes greater amounts of antioxidants to protect your skin cells than food alone can provide. But the story doesn't end there. Healthy skin also needs higher concentrations of vitamins and minerals for skin appearance and texture to reach its maximum genetic potential. In fact, various types of skin lesions, complexion issues, and skin conditions are aggravated by, or are the direct result of, an insufficient intake of certain vitamins or minerals. Fortunately, many skin problems clear up entirely within weeks of starting the right supplementation program. A high-potency multivitamin and mineral supplement must provide not only optimal levels of antioxidant nutrients, but also necessary levels of B vitamins, vitamins A and D, and other vitamins and minerals that help make the skin soft, smooth, radiant, and free of unsightly lesions.

B Vitamins and Skin Health

Virtually all B vitamins are required at sufficient dosages to ensure healthy development of skin cells. In fact, deficiencies in many B vitamins directly result in various types of skin conditions, skin diseases, and alterations in the normal appearance of the skin. Even marginal deficiencies of B vitamins can produce chronic skin lesions that are not treatable with topical agents alone. For instance, low intake of various B vitamins—such as vitamins B_2, B_3 or niacin, and B_6—is known to cause a condition called nasolabial seborrhea, which results in scaly, flaky, greasy skin where the sides of the nose meet the cheeks. A condition known as hyperpigmentation, in which the color of certain areas of the skin changes first to red, then to brown, can result from insufficient intake of niacin, folic acid, or vitamin B_{12}.

A marginal deficiency of vitamins B_2, B_3, and B_6, or iron is usually the cause of angular stomatitis, with symptoms of redness, cracking, and flaking of the skin at the corners of the mouth. Supplementation with a product that provides a B-50 complex (which means it contains 50 mg of most B vitamins along with 400 mcg folic acid, 50 mcg vitamin B_{12}, and 300 mcg biotin), and 5 to 8 mg of iron reverses these problems and prevents their recurrence. B vitamin supplementation has also been proven as an essential part of the nutrition and supplementation plan required to combat acne, eczema, and psoriasis.

B Vitamins for Smooth Skin

As noted in Chapter 1, vitamins B_2 and B_6 also work as helpers or cofactors in the synthesis of the good prostaglandin hormones PG-1 and PG-3 that largely determine the smoothness and texture of the skin. More recently, niacin (vitamin B_3) has been shown to help prevent skin damage induced by sunlight, known as photo-aging, by increasing the ability of skin cells to

My Success Story

MY SUCCESS STORY STARTED during my professional training in 1977 when I was in my early twenties. From the time I was a teenager, I had acne to a moderate degree on my face, shoulders, and upper back. There is nothing like a bunch of pimples on your face to knock the heck out of your self-esteem at that or any age. As part of my professional training, I received a full-year course in nutrition and another half-year course during my final year as an intern. Several years later, I went back to school part-time to complete a master's degree in science, with specialties in human nutrition and biology, but it was those first two courses in nutrition that sparked my interest and prompted me to see if I could find nutritional research to help solve my acne condition. I searched high and low for any published data, and it didn't take long to discover that several preliminary trials showed the use of certain vitamin and mineral supplements to be effective in reducing the severity of acne in a number of cases. Based on the research available at the time, I put together my own supplementation program of vitamins and minerals and began taking them every day.

Based on what I know today, my original program was actually elementary and incomplete. But it was good enough to reduce my acne by about 30 to 40 percent. And whenever I ran out of supplements and became lazy about replenishing them, my acne condition returned almost immediately, becoming increasingly severe. My girlfriend at the time would ask if I had stopped taking my supplements because she noticed the escalation of breakouts on my face. Although my dermatologist told me that nutrition had no effect on my acne, I was able to demonstrate that by "feeding" my skin cells with optimal levels of certain vitamins and minerals, I could improve my condition to a significant degree.

Though that was many years ago, it impressed upon me at an early stage in my career as a health professional that skin conditions can be influenced by diet and nutritional supplementation. So when patients ask me about their eczema, psoriasis, or other skin problems, I'm always willing to look for research that could provide an important missing link in managing their condition.

repair free-radical damage and by helping to preserve the cells' immune function. These experiments suggest that vitamin B_3 supplementation is involved in slowing the process of skin aging from UV-light exposure over our lifetime and may be an important aspect in preventing cancerous changes in skin cells.

We're Not Taking Enough B Vitamins

Data from the National Health and Nutrition Examination Survey II revealed that as a daily average, 80 percent of Americans consume less than the recommended daily allowance (RDA) for vitamin B_6, 45 percent consume less than the RDA for vitamin B_1, 34 percent consume less than the RDA for vitamins B_2 and B_{12}, and 33 percent consume less than the RDA for vitamin B_3. To make matters worse, the RDA values were not designed to represent optimal intake levels, but rather levels to guard against deficiency. Therefore, the RDAs are by no means the levels needed to maximize health and protect against degenerative and age-related diseases.

Taking a daily B-50 complex vitamin should be considered an important strategy to enhance and maintain the healthy appearance and texture of the skin. It also aids in the treatment of various skin conditions, as noted above, and prevents the development of B vitamin deficiency and insufficiency states that produce skin lesions.

Skin Cell Maturation: The Importance of Vitamins A and D

Normal growth and development of skin cells also depends on the influence of nutrients that promote the maturation of developing skin cells into fully developed adult cells prior to their arrival at the skin's surface. The transformation process that these immature cells undergo at the deeper layers of the epidermis before maturing into fully adult skin cells depends largely upon levels of vitamins A and D and beta-carotene.

We All Need Vitamin A Supplementation

Skin cells are known to require sufficient amounts of vitamin A to reach maturity and for the normal production of mucus and other secretions that keep surface tissues moist and resistant to infection. The National Health and Nutrition Examination Survey II demonstrated that vitamin A consumption across the U.S. population is of concern, with 50 percent of adult Americans taking in less than the RDA for vitamin A each day. In the absence of adequate vitamin A, the cells that line the passages of the mouth, throat, and stomach and the skin cells do not develop normally, nor do they produce normal secretions. Instead, these cells become covered or filled with keratin—the dry, water-insoluble protein we learned about in Chapter 1. Taking a daily multivitamin that contains 2,500 to 3,000 IU vitamin A and 10,000 to 12,000 IU beta-carotene helps support skin health and appearance and combats the high prevalence of vitamin A insufficiency, which contributes to skin complexion and texture problems and aggravates a host of skin disorders.

Additionally, vitamin A deficiency can cause a precancerous condition known as metaplasia in various cells that line the body's passageways and result in severely cracked, dry, peeling, and inflamed skin. The affected cells appear grossly enlarged and seem highly irregular and abnormal upon microscopic examination.

What's more common are cases of insufficient vitamin A intake, which aggravates skin problems like acne and disrupts the normal development and maturity of skin cells, lessening the smoothness and moistness of the skin. As a rule, supplementation with 2,500 IU vitamin A is all that is required to correct the insufficiency. Indeed, taking too much of the vitamin can be dangerous, because dosages above 5,000 IU a day can result in vitamin A toxicity over time. This level of intake can also cause severe birth defects in the offspring of women taking such high dosages. It's important to make sure the daily supplement you take contains no more than 2,500 to 3,000 IU vitamin A. In fact, in cases of vitamin A insufficiency, the body can manufacture the vitamin from beta-carotene, which should be supplied at 10,000 IU daily. Beta-carotene is nontoxic and can be taken safely at higher doses.

All this being said, however, there are some cases in which doctors will prescribe higher than the recommended dosages of vitamin A. For instance, vitamin A supplementation has been proven beneficial in wound healing, as it stimulates the synthesis of collagen. In such cases, physicians may recommend short-term supplementation with 25,000 to 50,000 IU vitamin A prior to and following surgery and various dermatological procedures to enhance healing and help ensure more complete healing of the skin and connective tissues. Dosages at these levels have also been used as a component of acne treatment. Still, it's important to remember that a medical physician must supervise this type of supplementation regimen due to the high risk of toxicity and associated birth defects.

Vitamin D's Role in Healthy Skin Cell Maturation

Skin cells also require vitamin D for their transformation from immature cells in the deeper layers of the epidermis into healthy, fully developed adult cells that will eventually reach the surface of the skin. Vitamin D slows the rate of cell division and turnover, thus acting as a preventive measure against cancer by guiding cell maturation away from malignant changes and toward normal adult cell development. It has been shown to prevent the onset of melanoma in experimental animal research, and has also been associated with a reduction in breast, prostate, and colon cancers. Recently it was discovered that most skin cells have vitamin D receptors, which indicates that skin cells depend on an adequate supply of the vitamin from the bloodstream to develop normally.

Vitamin D is also important for calcium absorption and is thus a key nutritional factor in the prevention of osteoporosis; a condition we will discus in greater detail in Chapter 7. Supplementation with the vitamin has also been proven helpful in the treatment of psoriasis by slowing skin cell division, which is excessive in psoriatic cases.

To promote general health and to enhance the amount of vitamin D available to skin cells, daily supplementation with 400 IU vitamin D is regarded as safe and effective and is the amount that should be contained in a well-formulated multivitamin product.

Northerners Need More Vitamin D

When sunlight hits your skin, it actually stimulates vitamin D synthesis in the skin layers. So a little sunlight exposure is actually a good thing. In fact, studies show that exposing your forearms to the sun for twenty to thirty minutes a day is all that is necessary to synthesize sufficient quantities of vitamin D.

Unfortunately, people living in the more northern areas of North America (above the 40th degree parallel) tend to have significantly lower levels of vitamin D in their bloodstream because they have less direct sunlight exposure on their skin year-round. In fact, their blood levels of vitamin D synthesized from the sunlight are often suboptimal from October to May. During these months, many Northerners require daily supplementation with 400 IU vitamin D from a high-potency multivitamin to reach vitamin D levels in the ideal range. Some people, however, may require additional supplementation up to 1,000 IU.

The Role of Minerals: Selenium, Zinc, Copper, Manganese, Magnesium, and Calcium

In addition to boosting antioxidant defenses within skin cells, a number of minerals are also vital nutrients for overall skin health and appearance. These include selenium, zinc, copper, manganese, magnesium, and calcium.

Laboratory studies reveal that selenium and zinc supplementation defends skin cells against free-radical damage from UV light. Selenium is required to activate glutathione peroxidase, an important antioxidant enzyme within skin cells. Without sufficient selenium intake, this enzyme is basically paralyzed and can't protect against attacks from free radical.

In addition to providing antioxidant protection as part of the glutathione peroxidase enzyme system, selenium also aids the production of PG-1 and PG-3, which make the skin softer and smoother. Studies show low blood levels of selenium are associated with both eczema and psoriasis. Selenium also strengthens the immune system and is considered an important anticancer nutrient.

Unfortunately, the typical North American diet contains only about 25 to 50 mcg per day of this important nutrient because many areas in North America have selenium-deficient soil. That means less selenium is passed along by plants up the food chain to the human diet. Studies strongly suggest that we should be deriving at least 100 to 200 mcg of selenium each day from a combination of diet and supplementation.

Zinc's nutritional contribution is necessary for oil gland function, local skin hormone activation, wound healing, control of skin inflammation, and regeneration of skin cells. Zinc supplementation has been used with success in the treatment of acne and as part of the nutritional treatment for psoriasis and eczema. Studies indicate that most adults consume only 8 to 9 mg daily of zinc from dietary sources, whereas the RDA for zinc is set at 15 mg.

For all these reasons, I recommend taking a multivitamin and mineral supplement that contains at least 100 mcg selenium and 15 mg zinc as part of a general wellness program for total body health and for the skin in particular. Higher levels of zinc may be helpful in cases of acne and other skin conditions, which will be discussed in Chapter 8.

Copper, manganese, and magnesium are required by skin cells to activate another important antioxidant enzyme called superoxide dismutase. This enzyme quenches and neutralizes what is known as the superoxide anion, a very damaging free radical created from sunlight. Additionally, copper and manganese are required to maintain the integrity of the connective tissue that provides strength and resilience to the skin, while magnesium supports the function of many enzyme reactions throughout the body, including skin cells. All of these nutrients are often marginally deficient in the diets of North Americans. As such, a good multivitamin and mineral supplement should provide 2 mg of copper, 5 mg of manganese, and 200 mg of magnesium.

Calcium is the most abundant mineral in the body. It makes up approximately 2 percent of body weight with 99 percent incorporated into hard tissues such as bones, teeth, and nails. The other 1 percent is contained in the bloodstream and within other body cells, where it participates in many important functions, including muscle contraction, nerve transmission, blood clotting, heartbeat regulation, and the secretion of some hormones. Calcium, zinc, and iron work synergistically to make nails smooth, hard, and resistant to breakage, peeling, and chipping.

Studies demonstrate that most people living in North America lack 500 to 800 mg calcium if their diet is to meet the daily recommendations set by the National Institutes of Health. As a result, our society is facing epidemic levels of osteoporosis as the population ages, with women over the age of fifty and men over the age of sixty-five facing hip and spinal fractures. That is one of the reasons I recommend taking a high-potency multivitamin and mineral supplement that contains 500 mg of elemental calcium and 400 IU of vitamin D, which is essential for calcium absorption. The role of calcium in the prevention of osteoporosis will be discussed in more detail in Chapter 7.

PREVENTING DAMAGE FROM FREE RADICALS

When it comes to free radicals and skin damage, there are two things you need to know. First, no matter how careful you are, during your lifetime your skin is going to suffer some damage from ultraviolet light exposure and other sources of free radicals, such as cigarette smoke and alcohol consumption. Second, to protect against free-radical damage, you must go above and beyond minimizing your exposure to UV light by reducing sun exposure to your skin, wearing protective clothing, and using proper sunscreen and suntan lotions. You must also protect your skin cells from free-radical damage from the inside-out, beyond what dietary measures alone can provide. You must take a high-potency, antioxidant-enriched multivitamin and mineral supplement every day of your life. Eating at least five servings of fruits and a day, containing many different antioxidants, is a prudent way to add more protection to your skin cells from dietary sources. It's also a well-accepted dietary strategy to help reduce the risk of many degenerative diseases.

This list summarizes what you've learned in this chapter:

- Free radicals cause extreme damage to our bodies, inflicting deep harm to skin cells, and lead to poor skin texture, premature aging and wrinkling, and even cancer.

- Free radicals are created when ultraviolet light penetrates the skin and injects oxygen molecules with a single electron. Now a free radical, the oxygen molecule begins searching for a second electron to neutralize itself. The free radicals steal electrons from surrounding molecules within the skin cell and, in the process, leave those molecules with only one electron, thereby creating more free radicals.

- Free radicals are also created by cigarette smoke and alcohol.

- Some of the premier nutritional antioxidants that protect the skin from the inside-out include vitamins C and E, beta-carotene, selenium, zinc, copper, magnesium, and manganese.

- B vitamins are also important for normal skin cell development. Many complexion problems and skin lesions are caused by insufficient consumption of B vitamins, which is a widespread problem in North America. A high-potency multivitamin and mineral supplement should include a B-50 complex, which provides skin cells with optimal levels of these important nutrients, improving skin texture and appearance and aiding in the treatment of various skin conditions.

- Vitamins A and D work synergistically to optimize the maturation of skin cells as they work their way up from the lowest layer of the epidermis to the top layer of the skin. Insufficient intake and synthesis of these two nutrients is prevalent in our society, and most people will benefit from taking a multivitamin and mineral supplement containing 2,500 to 3,000 IU vitamin A, 10,000 to 12,000 IU beta-carotene, and 400 IU vitamin D.

The following list shows the recommended high-potency multivitamin formula (see Resources). (Two caplets twice a day is the suggested dosage.)

Amount in 4 Caplets of the Recommended
High-Potency Multivitamin Formula

Beta-carotene	10,000 IU	Niacin	50 mg
Biotin	300 mcg	Pantothenic acid	50 mg
Calcium	500 mg	Selenium	100 mcg
Chromium	50 mcg	Vitamin A	2,500 IU
Citrus bioflavonoids	50 mg	Vitamin B_1	50 mg
Copper	2 mg	Vitamin B_2	50 mg
Folic acid	400 mcg	Vitamin B_6	50 mg
Iron	6 mg	Vitamin B_{12}	50 mcg
Lutein (5%)	6 mg	Vitamin C	1,000 mg
Lycopene (5%)	6 mg	Vitamin D	400 IU
Magnesium	200 mg	Vitamin E (all natural)	400 IU
Manganese	5 mg	Zinc	15 mg
Molybdenum	50 mcg		

Encapsulated Hyaluronic Acid: The Topical Essential Nutrient for Ageless Skin and Reversal of Wrinkles

Up to this point, we've explored a concept that is gaining acceptance, yet is still very foreign to many people: A clear, radiant complexion starts with healthy skin, and healthy skin begins within and works from the inside-out. That's why we've spent so much time learning about the skin, its functions, and the diet and nutritional supplementation you need to reach your goal of vibrant, healthy skin.

Now we're going to change direction and discuss a topical nutritional supplement—a solution applied to the skin—that is proven to reverse fine lines, crow's feet, and shallow wrinkles. Used in conjunction with the essential oils and the vitamin and mineral supplements, this topical solution takes skin smoothness to a whole new level that you may have thought impossible. How? The secret ingredient is a remarkable and vital nutrient called hyaluronic acid (HA). You're going to be very excited about how HA can help you reach your goal of outstanding skin.

HA IS AN ESSENTIAL NUTRIENT

Hyaluronic acid is a substance that's naturally produced by your skin cells throughout your lifetime. HA is a conditionally essential nutrient, meaning that it's more abundant in your skin when you're younger, and it functions to keep skin youthful, smooth, toned, and moist. A natural humectant (a substance that provides a moistening effect), the nutrient acts like an unbelievably thirsty little sponge. In fact, it holds up to 1,000 times its weight in water within the skin layers. The abundance of moisture HA can hold accounts for its amazing ability to make your skin feel really beautiful. By softening fine lines and superficial wrinkles, this remarkable nutrient can generally reduce and, to a significant degree, reverse the aging appearance of the skin.

HA DECLINES AS WE AGE

Our bodies begin to produce HA at a great rate from the day we're born. If you ever wondered why babies have such soft, supple skin, it's because their skin is super-enriched with hyaluronic acid. It's all downhill from there, though. With age, the body's HA production decreases, causing skin dehydration from the inside-out and contributing to skin aging. Dehydration leads to thinning of the skin; promotes the development of wrinkles, fine lines, and crow's feet; and generally makes the skin feel drier. By age fifty, it's estimated that we produce less than half of the HA we did in our youth. The decline in HA production that occurs as we age is a large reason for the decreased suppleness, reduced elasticity, and loss of skin tone we experience over time.

The key to keeping the skin in great condition throughout your lifetime is to feed it HA every day after about the age of twenty. You may find it reassuring to know that you can replenish your skin levels of HA back to more youthful concentrations by applying a topical HA serum every morning and evening. Supplementing HA in any other form is not effective because the body requires a substance called glucosamine to manufacture its own HA. However, even taking glucosamine supplements, which is helpful in restoring joint cartilage, has not been shown to increase skin levels of HA. The only reliable way to slow skin aging and to reverse fine lines, shallow wrinkles, and crow's feet is to replenish levels of HA in the skin through a topical application.

HOW DOES HA WORK?

Under ideal conditions, HA is found in all the layers of the epidermis and the dermis. It is actually retained between skin cells and forms part of the substance that holds cells together, very similar to the way mortar holds bricks together in a house. The difference is that HA doesn't simply provide structural support within the skin, but it also holds moisture within the skin, plumping it up to resist—or reduce and reverse—the formation of wrinkles. On the surface of the skin, HA acts as nature's most effective moisturizer. After the first few applications, you will begin to see some of the fine lines on your face disappear and the surface of your skin will feel smoother and silkier. But there's one hitch: You must use a form of HA that can be efficiently absorbed through all the skin layers. Not all HA products are formulated to this standard, and there's no sense spending your money on a cheap imitation that doesn't deliver.

The right HA product helps to maintain water balance in the dermis, while supporting the other dermal components, elastin and collagen fibers. HA is the medium through which epidermal cells must pass as they work their way to the skin's surface and take their place on the front line. In the process, HA provides developing skin cells with nutrients as they pass through the layers, directly supporting their metabolism, growth, and maturation.

HA also acts as a powerful antioxidant in the skin. Like some of the nutritional supplements taken orally, it helps prevent or minimize free-radical damage to the skin from sunlight and other sources of ultraviolet light that cause wrinkles, accelerated skin aging, and skin cancer.

HOW ENCAPSULATED ULTRAPURE HA WORKS

The key to making hyaluronic acid work to the best of its ability, so it can be distributed effectively throughout all the layers of the skin, is how it's delivered to the skin's surface. In its free form, HA is not absorbed very well by the skin, and it's too large to penetrate to the deeper skin layers with topical application. This and other properties restrict its absorption.

You can imagine how pleased I was when, during my research, I came across a method that provides the most effective HA topical delivery system. I found that HA must be surrounded by a special delivery agent called a second-generation liposome. Studies show that this encapsulated form of ultrapure HA is the most reliable, proven method to distribute the HA throughout all layers of the skin.

Here's what happens when HA is delivered to the skin's surface through the second-generation liposome carrier: Hyaluronic acid is formed from repeating linkages of two different sugar molecules so it's possible to make short and long chains. On a scale too small for the human eye to see, the HA arrives in a wide range of chain lengths—some long, some short. Since the longer chains are too large to penetrate the skin to any real depth, they remain at or near the surface. Instantly upon application, they begin to moisturize the skin's surface, making it look and feel smoother. Meanwhile, the shorter chain lengths are absorbed and work their way down to the lower levels of the skin to start hydrating the deeper layers of the epidermis and the dermis. Combined, these two steps give the surface of the skin a smooth, attractive appearance and, at the same time, enable the deeper layers to trap water molecules, plumping up the skin and giving it a more supple, elastic, and toned look.

Clinical trials and experimental studies have shown that with continued use, this ultrapure encapsulated form of HA reverses fine lines and wrinkles, crow's feet, skin aging, sagging, and loss of skin tone by acting as a natural filler. Results are often seen within the first two months of daily use.

A placebo-controlled study conducted in 1998 on healthy human volunteers demonstrated that this encapsulated form of HA is capable of both preventing and diminishing wrinkles, improving skin elasticity, and restoring the structure and organization of the collagen protein within the dermis. Experimental laboratory studies have also provided evidence that ultrapure encapsulated HA penetrates to all skin layers and produces a range of anti-aging effects on the skin.

HA PROMOTES HEALING

In addition to all the other remarkable effects it has shown, hyaluronic acid promotes wound healing. When HA penetrates your skin, it invigorates fibroblasts, cells that play an important part in the wound-healing process. When activated, fibroblasts within the skin secrete collagen and elastin, which provide the dermis with its strength, tone, and elasticity and are also key in healing. It should be noted that fibroblasts normally decrease in number and activity as we age. Topical HA basically reverses that process, encouraging fibroblast activity to function at the same level as in our youth. Thus, daily applications of HA also prevent the normal degree of age-related decline in skin collagen and elastin fibers.

HA has been used therapeutically to treat acute and chronic conditions such as abrasions, postoperative incisions, first- and second-degree burns, vascular and metabolic ulcers, and pressure sores. It has also been effective in reducing the incidence and severity of an inflammation of skin cells called radio-epithelitis, which commonly occurs in patients undergoing radiotherapy for cancer and other conditions.

THE IMPORTANCE OF A NONANIMAL SOURCE OF HA

As a topical nutritional supplement, hyaluronic acid is derived or synthesized from one of two sources: animal tissues or bacterial fermentation. I favor the

---

Success Story

Miss C Is Thrilled to Look Younger

Miss C was a thirty-six-year-old principal of an elementary school when she became curious about skin-care management and nutrition. For most of her life she had lived in a warm, sunny climate and had spent a great deal of time participating in outdoor sports and activities. Concerned that the many years out of doors had exposed her skin to cumulative damage from the sun, she was interested in preventing wrinkles and making her skin look more youthful naturally. After she was given a scientific explanation about how the program worked, she was willing to try the recommended high-potency multivitamin and mineral formula and essential oils supplement.

In less than a month, Miss C reported that her skin had become softer, smoother, and more radiant than she had ever before experienced. Having soft skin to begin with, she was delighted and amazed that it had become even more elegant. Then she began applying the encapsulated HA topical spray and serum on her face each morning and evening. Again, in less than a month, she reported amazing results. Fine lines on her face disappeared, and her overall facial complexion improved. How astonished she was to see that day after day, the sun-induced fine lines around her eyes were slowly disappearing and her face was beginning to look more youthful.

In fact, when school started in the fall, Miss C reported that many of the teachers (most of whom were younger) commented that she looked younger and her complexion was more sparkling than the last time they had seen her. She told me, "Even some of the parents of the children attending our school have been going out of their way to tell me how youthful I look. I haven't experienced anything like that in the past."

---

latter, as I believe it is a cleaner version of HA. Indeed, the animal-based source may be more susceptible to a wide variety of contaminants, including protein derivatives, which may trigger an allergic reaction or local tissue irritation. HA from animal sources may also contain heavy metals such as mercury, lead, or aluminum, which can travel through the bloodstream after being absorbed through the skin and from deposits in various tissues and organs. For your safety, the only type of HA that you should consider is the one supported by clinical studies—the ultrapure nonanimal-based encapsulated form (see Resources).

Success Story
My Office Staff

When I first became aware of the research related to ultrapure encapsulated HA, I ordered some of the product to try it out. At the same time, my office staff became curious about HA after I discussed the existing research with them and told them I was planning to use it. With that endorsement, the five female employees on the staff asked for the opportunity to test it out, too.

During the next two months, all five employees reported fabulous success stories. One forty-five-year-old told me she was hooked on HA after the first application, because she immediately noticed the reversal of fine lines and a more elegant look and feel to her skin. Soon after she started using HA, her friends commented that her skin looked more radiant and asked if she was doing something new. She described how HA worked and encouraged her esthetician to carry it in her salon. Since then, all her friends have begun using HA, as well as starting on the vitamin, mineral, and essential fatty acid supplement plan.

Another employee, a forty-six-year-old, noticed a marked improvement when the fine lines around her eyes and mouth disappeared within the first two weeks of using HA. She no longer needs to use an additional moisturizer. The other three staff members, who ranged in age from thirty-five to fifty-three, were also pleased to find that when they used HA in conjunction with nutritional supplements, the fine lines, crow's feet, and shallow wrinkles they had seen on their faces began to disappear. Plus, they noticed a more radiant complexion and softer, smoother skin—with little or no moisturizer.

I also noticed impressive changes as the fine lines around my eyes disappeared and my skin became more radiant. Other people did too, including my office staff. Neither I nor my staff will give up our HA regime any time soon!

SUMMARY: THE ROLE HA PLAYS IN PREVENTING SKIN AGING

Hyaluronic acid is a natural substance produced by skin cells and is found in great abundance in young skin. As a natural humectant (a substance that provides a moistening effect), HA binds to water molecules, holding up to 1,000 times its weight in moisture. That accounts for its amazing ability to keep the skin youthful, elastic, and supple, and to fill in fine lines and superficial wrinkles—reversing the aging appearance of the skin.

In the aging process, skin cells lose their ability to synthesize optimal amounts of HA, significantly contributing to skin aging. By age fifty, people are estimated to have less than half of the hyaluronic acid contained in their skin cells in their youth.

Clinical and experimental studies show that the topical application of a specialized blend of ultrapure encapsulated hyaluronic acid delivers the natural filler through all skin layers, including the deepest layers of the dermis. This unique carrier system has been the only proven, reliable method of delivering HA to all skin layers. Experimental and human clinical studies have demonstrated the effectiveness of this unique system of HA delivery. In one study, significant objective and subjective changes to the skin were observed during fifty-six days of regular daily use compared with a placebo. A recent human study demonstrated that HA delivered in the ultrapure form reversed fine lines, crow's feet, and shallow wrinkles within only two months of daily use. Upon application, it immediately improved the smoothness and appearance of the skin, and with continued use, more significant and lasting changes were seen, as HA concentrated and exerted its natural physiological effects throughout all skin layers.

Hyaluronic acid is also an antioxidant, so it can help prevent free-radical damage to the skin from sunlight, tanning beds, and other sources of ultraviolet light, as well as other sources of free radicals.

As an integral part of a comprehensive Wrinkle-Free Zone Program, everyone over twenty years of age requires HA topical application twice a day—in the morning and at night. Supplementing with this essential nutrient will enable you to:

1. Slow skin aging and prevent dehydration and the resulting fine lines and wrinkles that would otherwise appear on the face and neck.

2. Lessen the appearance of existing crow's feet around the eyes.

3. Enhance the moisturizing and hydration of the skin.

4. Make your skin look and feel smoother and more elegant.

5. Aid the healing of the skin wounds.

6. Help heal eczema lesions (HA serum should be applied directly to the lesions two to three times daily).

CHAPTER 4

The First Secret of a Clear Complexion: The Essential Role of Nutritional Detoxification

In recent years, skin-care professionals have begun to recognize just how important good nutrition and nutritional supplements are in preventing and controlling various skin conditions and complexion problems. They are beginning to understand the valuable role these substances play in producing the best in skin health and total body wellness.

The old adage "you are what you eat" is proving to be true. Many scientific studies have shown that a number of common skin conditions, such as psoriasis, eczema, rosacea, seborrheic dermatitis, and even acne can be improved by changing diet and supplementing with important nutrients for skin health. Although dietary modifications and the use of certain nutritional supplements may not totally resolve these skin conditions in every case, clinical studies and my own personal observations of patients and clients have shown that nutrition and supplementation can significantly improve these problems for a large number of people. My experience suggests that eczema, rosacea, and seborrhea are most responsive to the nutrition and supplementation program discussed in this book, whereas cases of psoriasis and severe acne are harder to predict. Mild to moderate cases of adolescent and adult acne tend to respond better than severe cases of adolescent and adult acne.

If you suffer from any of these skin conditions, I strongly suggest you incorporate the nutrition and supplementation program I will outline in this and the next two chapters into the global management of your condition. In most instances, moderate to dramatic improvement will occur, though some cases may be less responsive. Unfortunately, it is impossible to predict in advance which individuals will derive the best results.

We've seen in the three previous chapters that skin health can be dramatically improved by changing diet and taking recommended amounts of essential oils, vitamins, minerals, and antioxidants. People plagued by a skin condition or a complexion problem, however, need to take special steps to address their situation. Let's begin with the vital role of nutritional detoxification, which has been shown to have a huge impact on many skin conditions and complexion problems.

WHY DETOXIFICATION IS ESSENTIAL

What our bodies eliminate is just as important as what we take in each day in our continuing struggle for healthy skin. Detoxification removes poisons or other harmful substances, or toxins, from the body. Think of detoxification as a good spring cleaning, except instead of your house, you're ridding your body of all the stuff it has collected and no longer needs.

Where do these toxins come from? Everyday the body is bombarded with pesticides, herbicides, artificial flavors, and other foreign substances. In order for the body to perform and function at its best, it needs to flush out these toxins continuously to prevent any buildup that may lead to unhealthy skin or illnesses such as cancer.

Skin conditions such as eczema, psoriasis, and acne, as well as skin lesions and poor complexion problems, can be directly caused or aggravated by impurities in the blood that trigger what are known as "immune inflammatory reactions." Our immune cells view unwanted agents—unfamiliar chemicals from the environment, environmental toxins, toxins produced by bacteria, and end products of metabolism—as foreign bodies, or antigens, and initiate an attack on these substances. This, in turn, produces skin reactions in sensitive individuals. An obvious example is the formation of hives, which develop on the skin after an individual eats a food—strawberries, for instance—that contains a substance to which he or she is allergic in some degree. The body's immune cells attack the antigen from the strawberries that is traveling through the bloodstream, and an immune inflammatory response occurs that appears as hives on the skin.

Studies now show that many other chronic skin conditions besides hives are tied to various types of immune inflammatory reactions. To varying degrees, eczema, psoriasis, rosacea, seborrhea, acne, poor complexion problems, and some inflammatory skin lesions are a manifestation of chronic immune inflammatory reactions that result from an abnormal buildup of impurities in the bloodstream. When this happens, the immune system musters an assault against the perceived enemy by firing chemical torpedoes in an attempt to destroy it. But the battle comes with some other casualties, as the inflammatory response causes side effects that can trigger the formation of skin lesions, contribute to complexion problems, and aggravate existing skin conditions such as those mentioned above.

HOW THE BUILDUP OF BLOOD TOXINS OCCURS

The buildup of toxins, end-products of metabolism, and other foreign compounds can result from overexposure to toxins and environmental chemicals or from a slowing down of the body's enzyme detoxification systems. Unfortunately, sluggish detoxification is often the culprit.

The body's ability to rid itself of impurities normally slows with age, but in some instances this slowing can occur in younger individuals and is usually a factor in those who show signs of poor complexion or who suffer from various skin disorders. It's believed that as detoxification slows with age, the risk of cancer increases, because greater concentrations of dangerous substances that are not purged from the body continue to circulate throughout the body. This can lead to cancerous mutations in the genetic material, increasing the risk of cancer substantially with every decade of life. In relation to skin care, sluggish detoxification results in more impurities in the bloodstream that can trigger immune inflammatory reactions, produce or aggravate skin conditions, and contribute to problems with poor complexion.

The good news is that certain dietary habits and specific nutritional supplements can stimulate your body's detoxification processes to function on a more youthful level. These dietary and supplementation plans, when applied with the recommendations made in Chapters 1 and 2, have been proven to combat cases of acne, eczema, rosacea, seborrhea, and even psoriasis. For example, published research shows that supplementation with the correct dosage and standardized grade of the natural herb milk thistle provides marked improvement in patients suffering from psoriasis, which is one of the most difficult skin conditions to manage. Human clinical trials have also shown that improving the ratio of friendly gut bacteria to unfriendly gut bacteria through nutritional supplementation significantly reduces cases of eczema. I have seen great success with the strategy of diet and supplementation, and many other nutritionists, naturopaths, and holistic practitioners report the same promising outcomes.

If you have a complexion problem or one of the skin conditions mentioned above, you can benefit from learning how to improve your body's detoxification capabilities to achieve a clearer complexion. The trick is to reduce the level of foreign substances entering your bloodstream from the environment that may trigger immune inflammatory reactions and, at the same time, enhance your body's ability to eliminate impurities with appropriate nutritional supplementation.

Ridding your system of impurities is key to resolving chronic skin conditions and complexion problems. Now it's time to learn how to keep your detoxification enzymes working at maximum efficiency every day of your life.

HOW DETOXIFICATION WORKS

Let's take a look at how the body's detoxification system works to limit impurities in the bloodstream. The center of detoxification is the liver, which filters out the majority of the body's toxins as blood flows through it. However, remnants of metabolism sometimes remain. These remnants are unwanted junk produced when the liver enzymes break down hormones, prostaglandins, and other natural body chemicals. If these impurities are not detoxified and eliminated properly, they continue to circulate through the bloodstream. Then your immune cells attack these foreign substances, triggering immune inflammatory reactions that can aggravate a host of skin conditions and contribute to poor complexion problems. So the objective is to get these toxins and end products of metabolism detoxified efficiently—mainly in the liver—and eliminate them from the body in a safe, nonhazardous form.

STEP 1. Toxins enter the liver via the bloodstream.   **STEP 2.** The liver neutralizes or detoxifies the majority of toxins.

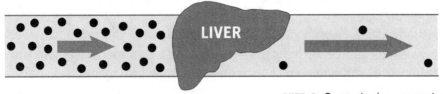

STEP 3. Some toxins are not neutralized by the liver.

FIGURE 4.1. Toxins that reenter the bloodstream can trigger skin inflammation.

Approximately 25 percent of the detoxification process occurs within the cells that line the intestines, while the other 75 percent or so takes place in the liver. Almost 2 quarts of blood pass through the liver to be detoxified every minute of your life. Any bacteria in the blood is captured and destroyed by extremely efficient, specialized immune cells called Kupffer cells located there. The Kupffer cells clean house effectively, killing 99 percent of the bacteria that get absorbed from the digestive system after a meal.

Detoxification of the end-products of metabolism, toxins, and foreign substances from the environment—pesticides, herbicides, food additives, and so on—that occurs in the liver cells takes place through a two-step process that we call phase I and phase II detoxification.

Phase I Detoxification

Phase I detoxification involves activating a group of enzymes called mixed function oxidase enzymes, clinically known as the cytochrome P450 system. This group includes 50 to 100 different types of enzymes whose only role is eliminate food colors, food preservatives, food additives, prescription and over-the-counter drugs, alcohol, caffeine, and other environmental toxins like pesticides and herbicides, collectively known as xenobiotics. Then one of two things happens. The first possibility is the toxins are completely neutralized, which rarely happens. The second, more common, outcome is not pleasant. More often than not, the toxins are converted into something more damaging than the form in which they arrived in the liver—free radicals.

Phase II Detoxification

Phase II detoxification enzymes interact with and neutralize the potentially damaging substances passed on from phase I and prepare them to be removed from the body. The enzymes do this primarily by attaching these dangerous compounds to a substance that neutralizes them and at the same time converting them into a form that the body can easily eliminate through the urine or feces.

In this manner, the phase I and phase II detoxification systems in the liver and intestinal cells work together to rid the body of harmful substances. Both phase I and phase II systems must be working at peak levels to prevent the buildup of toxic byproducts that may otherwise remain in the bloodstream and trigger immune inflammatory reactions that adversely affect the appearance of your skin.

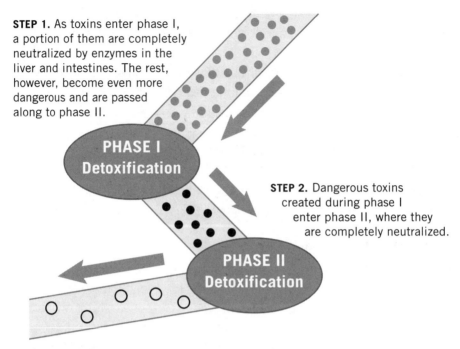

STEP 1. As toxins enter phase I, a portion of them are completely neutralized by enzymes in the liver and intestines. The rest, however, become even more dangerous and are passed along to phase II.

STEP 2. Dangerous toxins created during phase I enter phase II, where they are completely neutralized.

STEP 3. After leaving phase II, the neutralized toxins move through the system and are eliminated from the body via urination or a bowel movement.

FIGURE 4.2. Detoxification is an essential daily function that works in two phases.

NUTRITION AND DETOXIFICATION

You can help your body's detoxification system function more efficiently through a healthy diet and nutritional supplementation. Both of these strategies should be mandatory components of your overall plan for treating many skin conditions and complexion problems. It's important to understand that the kind of detoxification needed is not a twice-a-year cleansing-detoxification program. Rather, it involves the moment-to-moment efficiency of detoxification enzymes found primarily in your liver cells and to a lesser degree in other tissues. Boosting the activity of these enzymes is essential to keeping your blood pure from the toxins and other impurities that can trigger immune inflammatory reactions, thereby aggravating skin conditions and complexion problems. Nutritional detoxification relies on the daily use of certain foods and supplements that help optimize the functioning of these vital detoxification enzymes. People with skin conditions and complexion problems should use these strategies every day, because skin problems are often related to sluggish detoxification processes. The foods and supplements that help turbocharge these detoxification enzymes are safe to use every day of your life.

Boosting Phase I Detox with Diet and Supplements

Certain nutritional factors have been shown to affect phase I detoxification enzymes. For instance, eating cabbage, cauliflower, broccoli, bok choy, and Brussels sprouts—all members of the cruciferous vegetable family—has been shown to bolster these vital enzymes. Cruciferous vegetables contain a substance known as indole-3-carbinol, which boosts both phase I and phase II systems. That is one of the reasons studies show that people who regularly consume cruciferous vegetables have a lower risk of breast, prostate, colon, and possibly other cancers. Quite simply, these people are better able to detoxify any cancer-causing free radicals that may be circulating through their bloodstreams. So it makes sense for all of us to consume at least one daily serving of a cruciferous vegetable for general health reasons.

People with complexion problems, as well as acne, rosacea, eczema, seborrhea, or psoriasis, are advised to take a supplement that contains a pure grade of indole-3-carbinol. Taking a concentrated supplement of 25 to 50 milligrams (mg) indole-3-carbinol twice daily boosts the liver's detoxification activity far beyond what food alone can accomplish. This added support is needed to help jumpstart problems with sluggish detoxification.

Other substances known to support and boost phase I detoxification enzymes include limonene (a flavonoid, or beneficial plant compound, found in oranges), soy extract, and soy foods. Therefore, I recommend eating an orange or drinking a glass of pure orange juice daily, and taking in at least one serving of a soy product—soy milk, tofu, soy nuts, miso soup, soy cheese—and at least one serving of a cruciferous vegetable per day.

Another way to encourage the formation of phase I detoxification enzymes is to eat low-fat sources of protein, such as chicken, turkey, fish, egg whites, and low-fat dairy products. Suboptimal protein intake can impair detoxification activities. Low-fat sources of protein have a very high efficiency ratio, meaning that they match the protein needs of the human body, and are also low in saturated fat and arachidonic acid. Take note that the white meat of chicken and turkey are much lower in fat than the dark meat, so it's best to eat skinned chicken and turkey breast and to avoid eating the legs as much as possible.

Support for Phase I Detoxification

Certain foods and supplements promote phase I detoxification.

FOOD	SUPPLEMENTS
• Cabbage, cauliflower, broccoli, bok choy, Brussels sprouts	• Niacin (vitamin B_3)
• Oranges	• Riboflavin (vitamin B_2)
• Chicken, turkey, fish	• Vitamin C
• Soy-based food products	
• Low-fat dairy products	

Supplementation with riboflavin (vitamin B_2), niacin (vitamin B_3), and vitamin C also turbo-charges detoxification enzymes. The daily dosages required to help optimize phase I enzymes are 50 mg riboflavin, 50 mg niacin and 1,000 mg vitamin C. These quantities are found in the high-potency multivitamin and mineral supplement described in Chapter 2.

Support for Phase II Detoxification

Phase II detoxification is enhanced by certain foods and supplements.

FOOD	SUPPLEMENTS
• Cabbage, cauliflower, broccoli, bok choy, Brussels sprouts	• High-potency multivitamin and mineral containing: 1,000 mg of vitamin C, 400 IU of vitamin E (all natural), 10,000–15,000 IU of beta-carotene, 2,500 IU of vitamin A, 75–200 mg of selenium, 15 mg of zinc, 25–75 mg of magnesium, and 5 mg of manganese
• Oranges	• Essential fatty acid supplements (borage, flaxseed, and fish oils)
• Soy-based food products	• Indole-3-carbinol, milk thistle, reishi mushroom extract, and astragalus

Boosting Phase II Detox with Diet and Supplements

During phase II detoxification, the partially detoxified and usually dangerous free-radical remnants passed on from phase I are confronted with six types of neutralizing agents, rendering them harmless and preparing them for excretion from the body through the urine or feces. These neutralizing agents include the following chemical compounds: glutathione; amino acids; methyl groups, which create methylation reactions; sulfur, involved in sulfation and sulfoxidation reactions; acetyl groups that set up acetylation reactions, and the attachment of certain compounds to glucuronic acid, which leads to glucuronidation reactions.

It is important to know that each of these six phase II neutralizing reactions can be enhanced by specific nutritional factors. That means people with skin conditions can help clear impurities from their bloodstreams by taking recommended amounts of nutrients to enhance the action of phase II detoxification enzymes.

Optimizing Glutathione Levels: A Premier Phase II Detoxification Pathway Linked to Psoriasis and Other Skin Problems

Studies show glutathione neutralizing reactions are a very important aspect of phase II detoxification, so it is highly desirable for all of us to maintain optimal glutathione levels throughout our lifetimes. The neutralizing action of glutathione in the liver is known to be enhanced by supplementation with the right dosages of vitamins B_6, C, and E and selenium. Simply by taking a high-potency multivitamin and mineral supplement that includes these nutrients in the dosages recommended in Chapter 2, you can boost glutathione detoxification.

The herb known as milk thistle contains a flavonoid compound called silymarin, which has also been shown to boost liver glutathione levels and provide other benefits that enhance the liver's overall detoxification capabilities. For instance, people with psoriasis often notice a significant improvement in their condition by supplementing their diet with the recommended dosage of standard grade milk thistle.

I do not advise taking glutathione supplements. Many studies have shown that they are poorly absorbed from the intestinal tract into the bloodstream. In rare instances, supplementation with N-acetyl cysteine, may provide some benefit by boosting glutathione levels in patients with severely compromised liver and immune function. However, this is a more medicinal product and has been associated with some risks, and its use is not recommended unless it is prescribed by a trained health professional who is familiar with your health history.

Supplements That Boost Other Phase II Detox Pathways

Here are examples of how nutritional factors and specific supplements can boost the performance of the other phase II detoxification reactions:

1. For adequate amino acid reactions, your protein nutritional status needs to be optimal, as protein is made up exclusively of amino acids. Most women tend to consume too little protein on a daily basis, which can compromise detoxification activity and create such adverse health effects as suboptimal lean mass, insufficient bone mass and weakened immunity. That's why I recommend women boost their daily intake of protein by consuming a protein shake mix (made from whey or soy protein) to help ensure optimal intake of these vital amino acids. A good protein shake should provide 20 to 25 grams of protein in one scoop. Most adults require 70 to 150 grams of protein daily based upon their body weight and activity level. An active individual requires 1.25 grams of protein for each kilogram he or she weighs (1 pound equals 2.2 kilograms, so divide your weight in pounds by 2.2 to find your weight in kilograms).

2. Phase II methylation reactions require optimal nutritional status of such B vitamins as folic acid, B_6, and B_{12}.

3. Sulfation reactions require adequate intake of the sulfur-containing amino acids cysteine and methionine and of the mineral molybdenum. A rich source of these amino acids is a whey protein shake mix.

4. Acetylation reactions require optimal nutritional status of such B vitamins as pantothenic acid, B_1, and B_2, as well as vitamin C.

5. Glucuronidation reactions are enhanced by the intake of oranges, which contain limonene.

This look at the body's detoxification system illustrates how vital it is for you to feed your body optimal amounts of all the nutrients the liver needs to continually cleanse the blood and keep it free from impurities that aggravate skin problems and increase the general risk of cancer and ill-health.

THE NUTRITION AND SUPPLEMENTATION STRATEGY FOR PEOPLE WITH SKIN CONDITIONS OR POOR COMPLEXIONS

My own clinical experience, along with scientific studies and experimental data, indicate that various skin conditions and complexion problems tend to result when the body's detoxification processes become compromised. Supporting the liver's detoxification system with good nutrition and specific nutritional supplements, especially B vitamins and antioxidants, improves the skin's appearance in cases of eczema, acne (where low glutathione levels are common), psoriasis, rosacea, and seborrheic dermatitis. However, I have found that people who suffer from these skin conditions may need even more nutritional support. Studies have shown that supplementation with milk thistle and indole-3-carbinol is crucial in boosting detoxification to clear the bloodstream of impurities. This research prompted me to develop a detoxifying booster supplement that includes dosages of milk thistle and indole-3 carbinol, as well as two immune system regulators—reishi mushroom extract and astragalus.

The strategy to help boost and optimize the liver's detoxification capabilities is quite simple. First, you need to take the kind of high-potency multivitamin and mineral formula described in Chapter 2 that provides the recommended dosages of antioxidants (vitamins C and E and selenium) known to boost liver detoxification and support liver glutathione levels. This formula also contains B vitamins and minerals such as molybdenum that support most of the phase II detoxification enzyme reactions. You must also include the essential oils supplement—a combination of flaxseed, borage, and fish oils—described in Chapter 1 for your body to make the prostaglandin hormones PG-1 and PG-3, which reduce inflammatory activity associated with many skin conditions.

Finally, be sure to take a combination herbal product that contains the correct dosages and standard grades of milk thistle, indole-3-carbinol, astragalus, and reishi mushroom extract.

Milk Thistle

The silymarin content of milk thistle has been shown to enhance overall liver detoxification function, boost liver glutathione levels, and repair some existing damage to liver cells that may have occurred from past viral infections, drugs, and alcohol. It can also help defend liver cells against damage from current alcohol or drug use.

Success Story
Miss N Eradicates Lifelong Acne

MISS N WAS A FORTY-FIVE-YEAR-OLD WOMAN who had suffered from a moderate degree of adult acne her entire life. The condition was most pronounced in the T-zone area of her face, across the forehead and down along the nose to the center of the chin. I started her on the nutritional supplement program I've described, including the high-potency multivitamin and mineral formula, the essential oils supplement, and the immune detoxification support supplement. At the end of a sixty-day trial, she reported that her acne was reduced by 80 percent and that the skin all over her body had become exceedingly soft and smooth. In fact, she told me, "At my mother's eighty-first birthday party the other day, my sister hugged me and was amazed at how soft and smooth my skin felt." Miss N also noted that her nails were growing faster, were stronger than they had been, and were no longer peeling as they had for as long as she could remember. She was quite amazed and pleased that she began to see these results in such a short period for the first time in her life.

Indole-3-carbinol

Indole-3-carbinol is a plant-based nutrient, derived from cruciferous vegetables, which is known to supercharge both the phase I and phase II detoxification systems in liver and intestinal cells.

Immune Regulators

Astragalus and reishi mushroom extract are two well-known immune system regulators widely used in Asia in cases where immune system function is compromised, such as cancer, HIV infection, and hepatitis, and when immune system function needs to be better balanced. Because liver detoxification function is so closely tied to immune function in the body, it is vitally important to support both systems in those who suffer from skin conditions and complexion problems. This way, detoxification is optimized and immune inflammatory reactions are minimized, resulting in a clearer, healthier complexion.

The herbal detoxifying supplement for those who have skin conditions and complexion problems consists of the following ingredients in standard grades and dosages. Each capsule contains:

1. Milk thistle: 150 mg (standardized to 80 percent silymarin content)

2. Indole-3-carbinol: 25 mg (97 percent grade)

3. Astragalus: 100 mg (2:1 grade)

4. Reishi mushroom extract: 30 mg (standardized to 10 percent polysaccharide content)

The recommended dosage of this supplement to achieve maximum benefits is three to four capsules taken daily. (See Resources.) People with psoriasis may also find it necessary to take a stand-alone milk thistle supplement daily that provides an additional 200 mg (standardized to 80 percent silymarin content). See Chapter 8 for a summary of the nutrition and supplement protocols recommended for each skin condition.

REDUCING IMPURITIES IN YOUR BLOODSTREAM

If you have eczema, acne, rosacea, psoriasis, seborrhea, a poor complexion, or problem skin of any kind, the recommendations in this chapter will eliminate or greatly reduce the amounts of impurities in your bloodstream that are likely contributing to these conditions by triggering immune inflammatory reactions. In most cases, people following the program notice a better complexion in the thirty to sixty days after putting these strategies to work. However, effectively managing these skin conditions to achieve the best possible complexion also requires another step: You must also reduce the formation of toxins your body is probably producing within your intestinal tract. The next chapter will teach you how to achieve this result.

Here is a summary of how sluggish detoxification processes can lead to skin conditions and poor complexion and how the nutrition and supplementation strategies discussed here will help to combat these problems:

1. Impurities in the bloodstream—including end-products of metabolism, pesticides, herbicides, food additives, and bacterial toxins—can trigger immune inflammatory reactions that cause or aggravate complexion problems and skin conditions like eczema, acne, psoriasis, and seborrhea.

2. People with skin conditions and complexion problems need to boost liver detoxification of foreign compounds in the bloodstream in order to purify the blood and reduce immune inflammatory reactions.

3. Bolstering phase I and phase II detoxification in the liver means supplementing the diet with a high-potency multivitamin and mineral to take in optimal levels of antioxidants, B vitamins, and the mineral molybdenum. Taking a combination herbal supplement that includes the correct dosages and standard grades of milk thistle, indole-3-carbinol, astragalus, and reishi mushroom extract is also advised. Milk thistle and indole-3-carbinol interact directly with the liver's detoxification enzymes to supercharge their activity. Astragalus and reishi mushroom extract are known immune system regulators that help tone down immune inflammatory responses.

4. Individuals with skin conditions and complexion problems should reduce their intake of animal fats as described in Chapter 1. This will reduce both arachidonic acid intake and the synthesis of PG-2, the prostaglandin hormone that aggravates skin inflammatory conditions, including eczema, psoriasis, acne, and seborrhea.

5. To increase the production of PG-1 and PG-3, take an essential oil supplement that contains flaxseed, borage, and fish oils at the dosages outlined at the end of Chapter 1. These prostaglandin hormones exert a desirable anti-inflammatory effect on the various skin conditions and promote healthy skin.

6. Both cruciferous vegetables and soy products contain specialized nutrients that boost the phase I and phase II detoxification systems of both the liver and intestines. Eating at least one daily serving of a cruciferous vegetable (broccoli, Brussels sprouts, cabbage, cauliflower, bok choy) as well as at least one daily serving of a soy-based food (tofu, miso soup, roasted soy nuts, soy-based veggie burgers, or protein shakes) can help achieve these results.

CHAPTER 5

The Second Secret of a Clear Complexion: The Skin-Gut Connection

As you learned in Chapter 4, an overstimulated immune system can cause or aggravate skin conditions or complexion problems. Fortunately, specific nutritional approaches and supplements can boost detoxification enzyme activity in the liver to help keep the bloodstream clear of impurities that trigger immune inflammatory reactions. But the story doesn't end there. We also know that impurities in the bloodstream can build up as a result of insufficient digestive enzyme secretion in the small intestine and too many "unfriendly" bacteria in the large intestine. When these problems occur, partially digested food matter and toxins secreted from unfriendly gut bacteria enter the bloodstream and trigger immune inflammatory reactions that cause or aggravate skin problems. Some clinical studies and my own experiences with patients have shown that people with rosacea, psoriasis, eczema, adult acne, and other complexion problems often must address these underlying problems, in addition to boosting detoxification activity.

The direct connection between the gut and the skin is often overlooked. In many skin conditions and complexion problems, toxins and undigested food matter are absorbed from the gut into the bloodstream, causing immune inflammatory reactions like antigen-antibody reactions. In an immune inflammatory reaction, certain immune cells identify that some kind of foreign substance is present in the bloodstream, such as partially digested food that leaks into the blood from the small intestine or toxins generated from unfriendly gut bacteria or pesticides. These immune cells then bind to the foreign substance and generate an all-out attack that creates an inflammatory response. A common side effect of these inflammatory reactions is a worsening of skin conditions or complexion problems. Therefore, reducing immune inflammatory reactions that can cause or aggravate skin conditions is therefore critical. One of the means to do this is to block the formation of toxins and foreign compounds in the digestive tract that may otherwise leak into the bloodstream.

Sound difficult? Not really, if you follow the simple steps in this chapter. In addition to boosting the body's detoxification systems to rid the bloodstream of impurities, as described in Chapter 4, people with various skin conditions and complexion problems need to include a specific nutritional supplement to address problems that arise in the digestive tract. Digestive enzymes and the prebiotics known as fructooligosaccharide (FOS) and inulin are critically important to the skin-gut relationship. Prebiotics are nutrients that not only help the friendly bacteria to grow in the large intestine, but that drive out the unfriendly bacteria there as well.

DIGESTIVE ENZYMES AND SKIN HEALTH

Let's look first at the upper portion of the digestive tract. In the digestion process, enzymes are the essential agents that break down food into its singular components so that they can be absorbed into the bloodstream. The vast majority of digestive enzymes are secreted by the pancreas and the cells that line the upper intestinal tract. Small quantities of digestive enzymes, such as amylase, lipase and pepsin, are produced in the saliva and stomach juices, but these substances do not factor significantly into the overall digestion of a meal or a snack, as most of the digestion takes place in the small intestine. The more powerful enzymes from the pancreas and small intestine work with hydrochloric acid secreted in the stomach to break down food so that it is more easily assimilated into the body.

Often in people with complexion problems and various skin conditions like adult acne, eczema, psoriasis, rosacea, and other inflammatory skin lesions, the body does not secrete or manufacture optimal amounts of digestive enzymes. That appears to be especially true for women. Partially digested food can lead to problems like postmeal bloating and other intestinal symptoms, but it spells more serious trouble for people with skin conditions and complexion problems. In those cases, some of the partially digested food, especially derivatives of protein digestion, can leak into the bloodstream and trigger the kind of immune inflammatory reactions that cause or aggravate skin eruptions.

To illustrate this point, imagine the components of food matter entering the small intestine from the stomach like a series of boxcars linked together on a railway track. Our digestive enzymes are designed to unlink the boxcars from each other so that the individual boxcars can pass through the intestinal wall and enter the bloodstream. Once in the bloodstream, they are used as part of the body's normal metabolism. However, if the boxcars are not unlinked (for example, three amino acids are still linked together) due to insufficient amounts of digestive enzymes, a series of two or three boxcars can enter the bloodstream. In this instance, the immune cells in the bloodstream perceive these linked boxcars to be foreign substances and launch an immune inflammatory attack. Some of the linked boxcars that remain in the intestinal tract attract water. This, in turn, causes bloating after a meal, a problem frequently noted in women with insufficient digestive enzyme secretion.

If you have a skin condition or poor complexion, more than likely part of the cause is your body's inability to completely digest the foods you eat. I strongly recommend that you take a high-potency, full-spectrum digestive enzyme, extracted from nonanimal-based sources, at your two largest meals each day to help your body break down the food you have eaten and prevent partially digested food from entering your bloodstream.

A LEAKY GUT ADDS TO THE PROBLEM

As if it weren't bad enough that people with skin problems are usually deficient in digestive enzymes, the situation can be compounded by a condition known as leaky gut syndrome, also called intestinal permeability. Leaky gut syndrome occurs when improperly digested food ferments in the intestines, producing toxic byproducts that irritate the intestinal lining so much they cause tiny tears. Over time, the intestinal "filter" becomes less effective and allows toxins and undigested food matter to leak into the bloodstream, leading to immune inflammatory reactions. Invariably, where the cells lining the intestinal tract have been damaged and are unable to secrete optimal amounts of digestive enzymes, people also tend to have leaky gut syndrome. Leaky gut problems can occur with a variety of different ailments, including giardiasis, which is a parasite-induced condition that destroys the cells lining the intestinal tract; cell damage from frequent use of nonsteroidal anti-inflammatory drugs like aspirin and ibuprofen; or from excess alcohol consumption; damage related to celiac and Crohn's disease; or in cases where there is an inborn defect resulting in insufficient lactase enzyme synthesis, known as lactose intolerance. With all these conditions, the use of digestive enzymes is virtually mandatory to ensure that food is completely broken down and to prevent partially digested food from leaking into the bloodstream.

However, you don't necessarily have to suffer from a serious health condition to have less-than-adequate levels of digestive enzymes. Over the course of a lifetime, the majority of people will eventually have to deal with this to a certain degree. There is now evidence that most of us show a trend toward reduced digestive enzyme concentrations as we age.

INSUFFICIENT VITAMIN AND MINERAL INTAKE CAN ADD TO LEAKY GUT PROBLEMS

Various agents, such as alcohol and anti-inflammatory drugs, can damage the gut wall and increase the likelihood that partially digested food matter will enter the bloodstream and trigger immune inflammatory reactions. Unbalanced or unhealthy diets can also lead to this problem because the cells lining the intestinal tract require optimal nutritional support in order to function properly. Because these cells are replaced every seven to fourteen days, a continual supply of vitamins, minerals, and other nutrients are necessary to ensure that new cells mature fully and can perform their necessary duties. Thus, even marginal vitamin and mineral deficiencies, that are so common in our society can interfere with the proper development and functioning of the cells that line the intestinal tract, resulting in a greater susceptibility to leaky gut syndrome. In addition to the direct benefits to your skin, taking the high-potency multivitamin and mineral supplement described in Chapter 2 also ensures that the cells lining your intestinal tract will be healthier and, therefore, less prone to leaky gut problems.

However, no vitamin and mineral supplement can completely stop the leakage of partially digested food into the bloodstream if a person doesn't produce adequate digestive enzymes. Invariably, some partially digested food will enter the bloodstream, setting off an inflammatory reaction that worsens different types of skin conditions. That is why the use of a high-potency, full-spectrum digestive enzyme is so crucial in these cases.

DIGESTIVE ENZYMES CAN ALSO CLEAR IMMUNE INFLAMMATORY REACTIONS DIRECTLY

German researchers have shown that not only does taking digestive enzyme supplements work in the intestinal tract to enhance digestion, but some digestive enzymes are also absorbed into the bloodstream where they exert anti-inflammatory effects, dissolving immune inflammatory complexes before they can aggravate skin problems and other inflammatory reactions. That explains why digestive enzyme supplementation has been proven beneficial in controlling many cases of arthritis and other joint inflammatory conditions. Not surprisingly, the same holds true for many skin conditions that are aggravated by immune reactions. So if you suffer from skin problems, you should include digestive enzyme supplementation in your overall treatment plan.

Take note that all digestive enzyme products are not created equal. The one you choose should be a high-potency, full-spectrum formula in which each capsule contains 300 milligrams (mg) of a high-quality blend of enzymes such as amylase, protease I, protease II, lactase, lipase, cellulase, maltase, and sucrase. Taking two capsules twice a day with your two largest meals ensures that all food matter will be broken down into singular component parts so the body can assimilate them without creating an immune inflammatory response.

PREBIOTICS: THE FINAL FRONTIER IN CLEARING YOUR COMPLEXION TROUBLES

While digestive enzymes are an important addition to any nutrition game plan for people with problem skin, prebiotics are the last piece of the puzzle when it comes to clearing your complexion and managing existing skin conditions. Prebiotics help to remove the unfriendly gut bacteria from the large intestine. Unfriendly bacteria secrete toxins into the blood that trigger immune inflammatory reactions and aggravate various skin conditions and complexion problems.

The bacterial concentrations in the large intestine, referred to as gut flora, are composed essentially of "friendly" and "unfriendly bacteria." The higher the ratio of friendly to unfriendly bacteria, the better off your skin will be. Prebiotics are a specialized and unique type of soluble dietary fiber that are preferred by friendly bacteria such as bifodobacteria and lactobacilli, which are welcome inhabitants of the large intestine. When friendly bacteria are supplied with prebiotics, they divide and multiply rapidly and, as a result, crowd out the unfriendly bacteria that produce toxins—those foreign invaders that lead to immune inflammatory reactions. Many people who suffer from skin problems have an imbalance in their ratio of friendly-to-unfriendly gut bacteria, which results in the production and absorption of large amounts of bacterial endotoxins into the bloodstream. This triggers immune inflammatory reactions that make skin conditions worse.

The Gut Flora and Dysbiosis

The normal gut flora of the large intestine contain at least 500 different species of bacteria. Many of these bacteria are friendly, aiding in elimination, detoxification, and immune regulation, and supporting other functions of the body. They also provide an important aspect of protection to the body by neutralizing, or detoxifying, certain compounds; modifying immune response to foreign substances known as antigens; and controlling inflammatory reactions, which may involve the skin. Under certain circumstances, however, the large bowel can become overrun with unfriendly bacteria and other undesirable microbes, such as yeast and fungi, that can adversely affect skin health. Unbalanced flora in the gut, including organisms that do not normally cause infection—for example, bacteria and some species of yeasts and protozoa—induce disease by producing toxins or altering the nutrition or immune response of the body. This state is known as dysbiosis.

Overuse of antibiotics by humans and in animals and poor dietary habits, such as consuming lots of animal fat and not much dietary fiber, contribute to the high incidence of dysbiosis in North America and many other developed countries. Unfriendly bacteria, as well as certain yeasts and fungi, have been shown to secrete various toxins that can leak into the bloodstream and trigger immune inflammatory reactions, causing or aggravating skin conditions. That is why it is so critical for those who suffer from eczema, acne, psoriasis, rosacea, seborrhea, and poor complexion problems to flush unfriendly bacteria and undesirable microbes out of the large bowel and reconstitute the bowel with friendly bacteria that have been shown to help improve skin conditions and complexion problems.

FOS and Inulin Corrects Dysbiosis and Improves Your Complexion

Supplementing the diet with the correct amounts of the prebiotics FOS and inulin fosters the growth and replication of things like *Lactobacillus acidophilus* and other friendly gut bacteria. When these friendly bacteria start multiplying, they crowd out the unfriendly gut bacteria and other undesirable microbes that can inhabit the large bowel. This, in turn, stops the production of endotoxins that set off immune inflammatory reactions and cause or aggravate eczema,

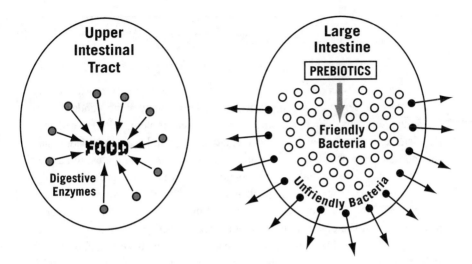

FIGURE 5.1. Digestive enzymes work in the upper intestinal tract to break down food so it can be easily absorbed into the bloodstream. When the prebiotics FOS and inulin enter the large intestine, they encourage the growth of friendly bacteria, which help detoxification, elimination, and regulation of the immune system. They also force out unfriendly bacteria.

psoriasis, acne, seborrhea, and rosacea. Simply put, higher concentrations of friendly gut bacteria—courtesy of prebiotic supplementation—make the gut a safer, healthier place, and help clear the bloodstream of impurities.

In addition, studies show that when FOS and inulin are taken to supplement the diet, the friendly gut bacteria replicate rapidly and exert a profound and favorable influence on detoxification, elimination, and immune system regulation. Taking prebiotics also reduces any tendency of the immune system to be overresponsive, as occurs in food hypersensitivity reactions that affect the skin. For example, clinical trials reported in *The American Journal of Clinical Nutrition* demonstrate that many cases of eczema can be completely resolved or significantly improved simply by modifying the concentrations of the friendly gut bacteria through supplementation.

The estimated average daily intake of FOS from food sources such as vegetables is 800 mg. Supplementation studies show that an additional 1,000 mg of FOS and inulin can favorably alter the bacteria populations of the large bowel. Therefore, to effectively combat skin conditions, 1,000 mg should be included in a supplement with high-potency, full-spectrum digestive enzymes, taken orally. (See Resources.) If you have a skin condition or poor complex-

---

Success Story
Miss K Overcomes Lifelong Acne

Miss K was a forty-eight-year-old school teacher who had suffered from acne since she was a teenager. Over the years, she had tried many of the standard medical acne treatments, which had failed to resolve her problem. With great skepticism, she agreed to follow the supplementation program I recommended, which included the high-potency multivitamin and mineral formula, the essential oils, the detoxifying booster, and the combination digestive enzyme-prebiotic.

After only sixty days, the blemishes on her back, shoulders, and face were reduced to a significant degree. She reported that this was the first summer in many years that she could wear a tank top because there were no lesions on her back, neck, or shoulders. She noticed that she was even getting fewer deep lesions, or cystic lesions, which not only are unattractive but can also be painful. Miss K stated that her nails were also stronger, while before they had been soft and had broken easily. Delighted to see such good results in such a short period of time, she continues to faithfully follow the supplementation regime.

---

ion, this combination enables you to address at the same time problems in both the upper and lower intestinal tract that are likely contributing to your symptoms. My experience shows various complexion problems clear up quickly when the combined supplement is used in conjunction with the detoxifying booster described in Chapter 4.

If you do not have a skin condition or a complexion problem, then you don't need to take this kind of combination product unless other health issues must be addressed. Keep in mind, however, that supplementation with prebiotics can also improve digestion and absorption of some nutrients, enhance detoxification by intestinal cells, reduce the concentrations of mutagens and carcinogens that are known to cause cancer in the large bowel, aid elimination processes, and favorably affect the immune system of the gut and the immune system as a whole. Positive effects on immunity include reduced hypersensitivity reactions to food and improved control of autoimmune conditions such as rheumatoid arthritis.

Probiotics Are Unreliable

I'm often asked about taking probiotics—friendly bacteria, such as *lactobacillus acidophilus* and *bifidus*—as an alternative to prebiotics. In clinically controlled studies, this approach has been successful, but in everyday life, it has proven to be an unreliable method of correcting dysbiosis. A number of consumer studies, reviewed at www.consumerlab.com, have shown that when probiotic supplements from retail outlets across the country are randomly sampled, virtually all the bacteria are already dead. This is because bacteria can only divide a finite number of times before the last generation dies. Once the bacteria are taken from the production facility's refrigerator, where they are stored at –50°C to stop them from dividing, they immediately begin to divide. By the time the bacteria are put into capsules, placed in a bottle, assembled with twelve bottles to a box, shipped to a storage warehouse, transferred to a regional distributor and transported to a retail store, so much time has elapsed that all the bacteria have usually divided for the final time. So taking probiotic supplements is a game of chance that may be unreliable because it is difficult to guarantee the number of live bacteria in probiotic products at the time you purchase them. Studies show taking

---

Success Story
Miss D Conquers Lifelong Acne

Miss D was a forty-four-year-old woman who'd had acne breakouts on her back and chest since she was a teenager. She was growing increasingly concerned about her aging skin and the damage caused by long-term smoking. After recommending standard health-promoting dietary and lifestyle modifications, I started Miss D on four of the skin supplements, including the high-potency multivitamin and mineral formula, the essential oils, the detoxifying booster, and the combination digestive enzyme prebiotic. I also included the encapsulated HA spray and serum.

Within a couple of months she reported the following changes:

- At least a 60 percent reduction in acne blemishes.

- Half the fine lines on her face had disappeared.

- Her skin was 100 percent softer and smoother, and its texture was significantly improved.

- Her fingernails were stronger and no longer curved or spooned, which can be an indication of iron insufficiency. The ridges on her thumbs and big toes—often a sign of calcium or vitamin D insufficiency—were reduced by 50 percent.

FOS and inulin is a more reliable method of increasing amounts of friendly gut bacteria.

Studies show that consuming yogurt and other soured and fermented foods that contain live bacterial cultures can support the growth of friendly bacteria. So I recommend that my clients and patients who suffer from skin conditions and complexion problems consume foods that contain live bacteria, such as yogurt, and take a supplement that contains prebiotics to help foster the growth of existing friendly gut bacteria and friendly bacteria from food sources.

Psoriasis and Bacterial Endotoxins: A Proven Link

To illustrate how unfriendly gut bacteria can contribute to skin conditions, let's look at one study that linked psoriasis with high levels of endotoxins circulating in the bloodstream from unfriendly gut bacteria circulating in their bloodstream. Patients with psoriasis showed significant reduction in psoriatic skin lesions when given a drug that binds to endotoxins in the large intestine, preventing the endotoxins from entering the bloodstream. While this treatment may be beneficial, the best approach is to force the unfriendly bacteria out of the large bowel so no endotoxins are formed in the first place. That's why I recommend that prebiotics be included with a digestive enzyme supplement.

Further proof that bacterial endotoxins aggravate psoriasis was noted in a study involving ninety-two patients taking a high-fiber supplement that binds to endotoxins in the gut. Within the patient group given the endotoxin-binding fiber, 62 percent showed marked reduction in the number of skin lesions, with all lesions in 18 percent of patients completely cleared. This is truly remarkable, as psoriasis is one of the most difficult skin problems to manage.

A personal story eloquently confirms the study outlined above. Not long ago I gave a presentation on nutrition and skin care to a group of estheticians as part of an educational day for skin-care professionals. As I explained the scientific aspects of how nutrition and supplementation should be included in the overall management of clients who had psoriasis and other skin conditions, I noticed out of the corner of my eye that the speaker to follow me was vigorously nodding her head in agreement with every statement I made. After my lecture, the woman started her presentation (on a topic completely unrelated to mine) by telling the audience that she had suffered from a severe form of psoriasis for many years. Out of desperation, when nothing else seemed to work, she started researching to see if any nutritional intervention could be of value. She told the audience that she had put into practice all the strategies I had just outlined and, within months, her problem was completely reversed and the psoriasis resolved. She noted that she had started using these nutrition and supplementation strategies many years ago, faithfully adhered to the practice, and the problem has never returned. The estheticians, only too well aware that psoriasis is a very difficult skin problem to conquer, listened almost in disbelief.

SUMMARY: CLEARING YOUR COMPLEXION

The development or aggravation of complexion problems, as well as condi-

Success Story
Miss BC Beats Psoriasis

Miss BC, a fifty-year-old woman, had recently developed a severe form of psoriasis on her hands and feet. Her family doctor had sent her to a dermatologist who told her little could be done to help such a severe case of psoriasis as hers. I noted that the lesions on her hands, fingers, and the bottom of her feet were so extensive and deep that blood was oozing from the skin in those areas. In tears she told me that she wasn't able to use her hands for even the simplest everyday tasks and that the lesions on her feet were so painful she could hardly walk.

I explained the connection between nutrition and supplementation and their effects on some cases of psoriasis. Willing to try anything that might help, Miss BC began the recommended daily supplementation protocol, taking the high-potency multivitamin and mineral formula, the essential oils, the immune-detoxification booster, and the full-spectrum digestive enzymes with prebiotics. Three weeks after beginning the program, Miss BC proudly showed me the dramatic improvement. Her hands and feet were at least 50 to 60 percent improved, with no more deep bleeding lesions. Feeling much better, she was able to get around more easily and could again use her hands again for all her basic lifestyle demands.

I had photographed Miss BC's hands and feet on her first visit, and did so again when she showed me the improvement in her condition. Using before and after pictures is very helpful to show doctors and estheticians how powerful supplementation can be to help manage psoriasis, which is one of the most stubborn skin conditions. Not all psoriasis cases will see such amazing results with changes in diet and use of a targeted supplementation program, but it's really rewarding when such a success story happens.

tions like eczema, psoriasis, acne, seborrhea, rosacea, and other inflammatory skin conditions, has been linked to sluggish detoxification processes and an increase in toxins or impurities in the bloodstream. Poor detoxification doesn't clear impurities from the body efficiently, while digestive enzyme insufficiency and intestinal dysbiosis may actually contribute to higher levels of toxins in the bloodstream. A comprehensive nutrition and supplementation strategy can help clear the bloodstream of impurities that trigger the immune inflammatory reactions that adversely affect the skin.

In addition to standard topical, or external, treatments for skin conditions, the following supplements should be incorporated into the overall management of these problems:

1. To support liver phase I and phase II detoxification, take a high-potency multivitamin and mineral supplement that is enriched with a B-50 complex and the following antioxidants:

   - Vitamin C: 1,000 mg

   - Vitamin E: 400 international units (IU), all natural

   - Beta-carotene: 10,000 to 15,000 IU

   - Selenium: 100 to 200 micrograms (mcg)

2. Include a daily immune-detox support supplement containing indole-3-carbinol, which is the active detoxifier in cruciferous vegetables, and milk thistle standardized to 80 percent silymarin content. For additional support, a product of this kind should also contain two powerful immune-modulating herbal components, reishi mushroom extract and astragalus, which are known to regulate immune function and minimize immune inflammatory reactions. A healthy immune system is associated with a healthy-looking complexion and enhances total-body wellness.

3. Eat at least one daily serving each of a cruciferous vegetable and a soy-based food product, as outlined in Chapter 4.

4. Include a daily shake in your diet that is rich in soy and whey protein, if you are not sensitive to them. Soy and whey proteins support amino acid interactions in the liver and strengthen both the immune system and the intestinal barrier to toxins. Soy isoflavones included in soy protein shakes also improve the performance of many phase II liver enzymes, making them more efficient.

5. To support intestinal tract detoxification, make sure to include fiber in your diet or take a fiber supplement each day, such as 2 teaspoons of psyllium husk fiber or 2 tablespoons of flaxseed powder. Fiber helps to clear out any bowel toxins and carcinogens.

6. If you have a skin condition, complexion problem, food sensitivity or allergy, or digestive disorder, or if you are prone to inflammatory reactions, take a daily supplement providing 700 mg of FOS and 300 mg of inulin in combination with high-potency, full-spectrum digestive enzymes. (See Resources.)

7. Take an essential oil supplement containing borage, flaxseed, and fish oils to increase the synthesis of PG-1 and PG-3, as these prostaglandin hormones decrease skin inflammation in cases of eczema, psoriasis, acne, rosacea, and seborrhea.

8. Be aware that PG-2 can aggravate skin conditions, so be sure to eat a diet that is low in animal fat to minimizes your intake of arachidonic acid.

9. Reduce your use of alcohol and drugs, and limit exposure to environmental agents known to damage the intestinal lining or suppress the growth of friendly gut bacteria.

   Nutritional support of intestinal tract health and liver detoxification is a vital but often neglected aspect of skin-care therapy and management. Such a course of action includes proven, effective, complementary strategies to help combat many chronic or recurrent skin problems. The time has come to recognize that nutrition and supplementation are essential components in preventing and treating various skin conditions; improving skin texture, moisture, and appearance; and minimizing or reversing the appearance of fine lines and wrinkles.

CHAPTER 6

Treating Acne, Rosacea, Chronic Fungal Infections, Psoriasis, and Eczema Using Oil of Oregano

There is one other key ingredient in the nutritional management of skin care that has remained closely guarded for centuries: oil of oregano. A high-potency grade of oil of oregano effectively kills bacteria on the skin that cause acne, as well as the skin mite associated with rosacea. It also kills fungal infections of the skin, which may affect the feet and toes of up to 40 percent of the patients seen by skin-care professionals.

Recent studies show that bacteria such as *Staphylococcus aureus* and streptococci are present in the skin lesions of psoriasis and eczema, where they promote inflammatory processes that aggravate these conditions. Some doctors have successfully treated cases of psoriasis and eczema with antibiotics that kill these bacteria in the skin and in the bloodstream. Unfortunately, long-term use of antibiotics comes with an extensive list of undesirable side effects, and therefore should be avoided as much as possible. In some cases, high-potency oil of oregano can be substituted for antibiotics, because it also kills these bacteria; as such, it is an important component in the treatment of psoriasis and eczema.

The wonderful news about oil of oregano is that both internal and external use is highly effective in treating and reversing acne, rosacea, and chronic fungal infections of the skin. It is also beneficial as an adjunctive intervention for psoriasis and eczema. More important, it does not cause the many undesirable side effects resulting from the use of antibiotics and harsh topical agents prescribed in conventional medicine for these skin disorders.

Let's take a closer look at these conditions so that we can better understand them and appreciate the unique and unprecedented role oil of oregano can play in helping to safely alleviate these problems.

CURING ACNE

Acne strikes terror into the hearts of most teenagers. They can pretty much handle all the other stuff that goes along with being that age—curfews, first loves, and occasionally being grounded—but as many as 80 percent of North American young people ranging in age from early teens to mid-twenties have met their match when it comes to acne vulgaris. Acne's prevalence has earned it notoriety as the most common skin disease among Americans and Canadians.

Because of increased testosterone levels, boys are more likely than girls to develop severe acne during their teenage years. Studies have concluded that only one out of three teenagers with acne seeks help for the condition, despite the fact that virtually everyone who suffers from it acknowledges that the problem affects their self-image.

The good news is that acne usually isn't permanent, and most people grow out of it. But the bad news is that there are exceptions. In fact, many people struggle with the effects of acne for many years. In serious cases, the skin can even be permanently damaged.

Acne Clogs Pores

The easiest way to help you understand how acne occurs is to think about a kitchen sink getting clogged, so water can't flow through it. As the water builds up in the sink, it starts to look pretty disgusting if you keep dumping dinner scraps and the like in there. Before long, you've got to grab the plunger and pour in drain cleanser to get out the debris.

With that picture in mind, imagine your body is the sink and the pores on the surface of your skin are the drains. To be able to operate efficiently and continually flush toxins and moisture from your body, the pores must be clear. If they're not, that's the first step toward developing acne.

Pores begin to clog when the body starts to produce excessive amounts of the oil sebum. This oil is secreted courtesy of the 5,000 sebaceous glands located throughout the body but mostly concentrated on the face, shoulders, upper arms, chest, and back. The sebaceous glands are big when we're born; then they shrink for a dozen years or so. In adolescents just on the edge of puberty, whose hormone levels are on the rise, the sebaceous glands kick back into action and begin producing oil at a rate that would be the envy of any member country of OPEC.

Oil from the sebaceous glands spreads on the skin and thickens as it comes into contact with dead cells, clogging the pores. Extensive medical research still has not been able to determine why a person's body suddenly begins to produce so much sebum, or why it is not able to flush away the dead cells with which the oil ultimately bonds. As a result, toxins that are usually flushed out start to build up in the body. Then, just when you thought it couldn't get any worse, along come *Propionibacterium acnes,* or *P. acnes* for short. This particular bacteria is found on the surface of everyone's skin, but it's present in greater concentrations in people whose bodies produce excess sebum because the bacteria feed off the oil, *P. acnes* bacteria, in combination with sebum and dead cells, cause inflammation in the hair follicles.

Excess oil plus dead skin cells and the *P. acnes* bacteria result in the inflammation and infectious process that cause pimples, whiteheads, and blackheads to form most commonly on the face, neck, and other areas of the body where sebaceous glands are concentrated. More serious pimples—deep, large pimples called cystic lesions—can result in painful infections and may even leave permanent scars.

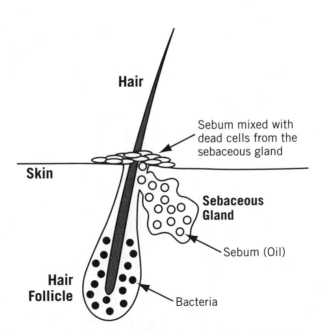

FIGURE 6.1. In the early teenage years, the sebaceous glands begin to produce great amounts of sebum (oil) and shed dead cells. The oil and dead cells combine into a thick substance that blocks hair follicles. Bacteria build up in the follicles, causing inflammation, leading to pimples, whiteheads, or blackheads.

A Range of Factors Can Cause Acne

There is also evidence that the pH of the skin, which reflects how acidic or alkaline the skin is, can affect developing acne. An acidic pH helps to keep pores clean and discourage bacteria buildup. Under normal conditions, the skin is naturally acidic. However, if the skin's pH balance shifts toward more alkaline, it can lead to potentially damaging bacterial activity.

People most at risk for this second scenario are those with raging hormones—teens and young adults. Hormonal changes that people in this age range experience may cause pH balance to swing from acidic to alkaline. With that switch comes a wide variety of unpleasant and unwanted microbes.

Additionally, certain types of medication have been known to stimulate acne in some people. If you are taking a prescription drug of any kind and you have acne, ask your physician or pharmacist if the particular drug could be contributing to your problem. In such cases, acne usually disappears when use of the medication is discontinued.

Another factor in the development of acne is genetic predisposition. It could just be that acne is coded in your genes—something else to which you owe your parents.

Finally, scientific studies suggest that some foods aggravate acne. These primarily include processed foods and ingredients, citrus fruit, refined vegetable oils, hydrogenated oils, deep-fried foods, caffeine, sugar, cocoa, chocolate, and nuts, to name just a few. However, there is still much debate about these nutritional influences. It's best to limit your intake of high-fat and fried foods, as well as sugary treats and chocolate products, as much as possible. As a teenager who once suffered from acne myself, I noticed that these foods tended to make my condition worse. In my early twenties, as a student of science,

---

Acne-Causing Foods

Avoiding these foods may help you avoid acne.

- Processed foods and ingredients
- Citrus fruits
- Refined vegetable oils
- Hydrogenated oils
- Deep-fried foods
- Caffeine
- Sugar and cocoa

I researched the relationship between nutrition and acne, and put together my own diet and supplementation program that reduced my acne condition by approximately 30 to 40 percent. (See "My Success Story" on page 35.)

Don't Make Acne Worse

Before starting any type of treatment, it is imperative not to aggravate acne, which can be irritated and made worse if tight clothing, straps, athletic equipment, and even scarves and turtleneck sweaters continually rub up against affected areas. As much as possible, areas of the body with acne should be clear of anything that might cause friction.

Even your best efforts at clearing up acne can aggravate the condition. Washing with a harsh soap, using very hot water, or even scrubbing too hard may make the problem worse. Just letting oily hair fall onto the forehead or cheeks feeds the *P. acne* bacteria. Excessive sweat and stress can also contribute to outbreaks.

Certain skin and hair products containing irritants should be avoided, especially oil-based products like milky cleansers, cold creams, lipsticks, and lip gloss. It's preferable to use special water-based skin-care products that gently cleanse the skin. A number of effective nonprescription medicated creams, soaps, lotions, and gels are on the market. Ask your doctor, esthetician, or dermatologist to recommend name brands available in your community.

Oregano to the Rescue

Hope and relief for acne sufferers comes from a powerful herb that grows high in the mountain meadows of certain regions in the Middle East, especially along the most easterly tip of the Mediterranean. Oil extracted from this highly potent variety of oregano has been proven effective in the treatment of acne because it contains antibiotic and anti-inflammatory properties that act as a one-two punch against the condition. The antibiotic action works to break down and kill the bacteria, while the oil's natural drying action shrinks and even dissolves acne lesions.

The reason the high-potency form of oil of oregano effectively kills acne is because it contains the volatile oils carvacrol and thymol, which carry the bulk of its antimicrobial and antifungal strength. Flavonoids and vitamins A and C are also found in this amazing medicinal product, and they work in unison with its other properties to fight a wide assortment of microscopic invaders, including acne-causing bacteria.

Does high-potency oil of oregano really work? For many people, it works like a charm. Original research by Dr. Cass Ingram, D.O., first made me aware of the multiple health benefits from the use of a high-potency oil of oregano supplement, as well as its topical application in cases of acne, rosacea, psoriasis, eczema, and fungal infections in the skin. Acknowledged by many as perhaps the world's leading expert on the use of oil of oregano, Dr. Ingram has conducted research and case studies that prompted me to recommend the form of oil of oregano that he used clinically with his own patients over the years with success.

You Need the Right Oil of Oregano for the Job

Not all oil of oregano supplements are created equal, however. Some of the hybrid species of oil of oregano have caused dangerous side effects when taken internally. The variety of oil of oregano researched and developed by Dr. Ingram is the best in the world because it contains the highest levels of active ingredients but is at the same time extremely nontoxic, safe, and effective. That is largely due to the perfect climatic conditions in the regions where this form of high-potency oregano grows naturally. For all of these reasons, I recommend only the oil of oregano produced by Dr. Ingram's group as part of my treatment regime for acne and other skin conditions.

Success Story
Miss M Gets Rid of Stress-Induced Acne

MISS M WAS A THIRTY-SIX-YEAR-OLD WOMAN who developed a moderate to severe case of adult acne that had been triggered by a stressful and tragic event the previous year. After trying numerous traditional approaches, she consulted me about nutritional supplementation, and I started her on the high-potency multivitamin and mineral formula, essential oils, and detoxifying booster supplements. But her condition persisted after a two-month trial. It is possible that stress had weakened her immune system and given the acne bacteria a green light to go to work on her skin, producing numerous blemishes on her face. After we added the high-potency oil of oregano product to her regime, she saw a difference in her complexion within the first two weeks. Hers was one of the first cases that convinced me of the need to include high-potency oil of oregano in any nutrition and supplementation game plan to combat acne.

Experts like Dr. Ingram attribute the success of oil of oregano to the high concentration and proper balance of its volatile oils. These provide the antiseptic effects so effective in killing undesirable bacteria, fungi, skin mites, and so on. Also of note is the fact that along with the plant's oil, oregano leaves and much of the dried herb have been used for medicinal purposes for many centuries.

I recommend that patients with acne take one to two capsules twice a day of the high-potency oil of oregano product. (See Resources.) Each capsule contains 450 milligrams (mg) of a proprietary blend of the wild high-mountain oregano herb loaded with the active ingredients that kill off the acne-causing bacteria. Oil of oregano cream should also be applied topically directly on acne lesions for overnight treatment. (See Resources.)

It's important to note that women who are pregnant should not take oil of oregano supplements, as they stimulate menstruation and could lead to miscarriage. Also, the topical application should not be used on mucous membranes in greater than a 1 percent concentration. Also, people with extremely sensitive skin should not use oregano oil topically, and it should never be used in treating children under two.

High-potency oil of oregano is an important product for overall treatment for acne. You will be amazed to see how effective this little-known and underappreciated natural treatment can be. Oil of oregano is a very safe product and has not been associated with any serious side effects or negative health outcomes in thousands of years of use when used responsibly.

Other Conventional Acne Treatments

Over-the-counter and prescription acne creams usually contain benzoyl peroxide, which indirectly releases free radicals that kill the acne-causing bacteria on the skin, thus preventing them from infecting the plugged sebaceous ducts. These helpful antibacterial creams have minimal side effects, such as dry, red, or itchy skin. However, taking antibiotics requires careful consideration. Though they are successful in preventing and treating new inflammatory lesions, they have little effect on existing lesions. Thus, it may require up to two months of therapy before positive results are seen. But the real issue here is the frequency and severity of side effects associated with antibiotic use. That is why I believe oil of oregano should be tried first.

Let's look at the side effects that can result from the indiscriminant use of antibiotics. First, antibiotics kill friendly gut bacteria, which can lead to prob-

Success Story
Master B Triumphs over Teenage Acne

Master B was a twenty-year-old student who had suffered from severe acne since he was age fifteen. His parents had spent $3,000 to $4,000 on microdermabrasion treatments and other procedures to help reduce the severity of his acne, and he'd had a couple of rounds of the antibiotic tetracycline to try to help his condition. But none of the solutions provided any lasting benefits, and the tetracycline made very little difference in his condition. I recommended that Master B begin supplementing with the high-potency multivitamin and mineral formula, the essential oils, the detoxifying booster, and the combination digestive enzyme-prebiotics. After following the program faithfully, he reported within the first two months that his acne condition had cleared up 90 percent—and that was before he started the high-potency oil of oregano supplement. Master B was thrilled with the results, has followed the program faithfully, and continues to be successful in his fight against acne.

lems with elimination, detoxification, and immune regulation, and increase susceptibility to infections in the intestinal tract. These problems, in turn, can lead to increased risk of inflammatory bowel disease and the development of antibiotic-resistant strains of bacteria that can cause infections no longer treatable with antibiotics.

The list doesn't end there. Other recorded effects include super-infections of the mouth, intestinal tract, rectum, or vagina from yeast organisms. Also associated with antibiotic use are symptoms such as intestinal upset and abdominal cramping; drug-induced hepatitis or jaundice; low platelet blood count, or anemia, which causes abnormal bleeding or bruising; tremors; and the activation of the autoimmune disease known as lupus. Plus, antibiotics may cause a serious skin rash when the skin is exposed to sunlight. Therefore, in the treatment of acne, antibiotics should not be your first choice for the treatment of acne if at all possible.

Using a high-potency oil of oregano supplement and topical cream is a safer, and in some cases a more effective, means to control acne. However, acne can be a stubborn condition to treat, so you should try a high-potency oil of oregano first, in conjunction with the rest of the nutrition and supplementation program summarized in Chapter 8. If your condition persists after sixty days of beginning supplementation, consult your doctor or dermatologist about taking antibiotics.

Vitamin and Mineral Supplements Also Fight Acne

Over the years, a number of studies have shown that supplementation with various vitamins and minerals that support skin health can improve acne conditions. I found that to be true in my own case when I was in my early twenties so, naturally, I have recommended these dietary and supplementation practices to my patients over the past twenty years. Studies have particularly highlighted the effectiveness of selenium, zinc, and vitamin A in treating acne. The scientific literature shows that selenium caused significant improvements in a study using a group of men and women with moderate to severe acne. In this instance, treatment included 200 micrograms (mcg) selenium in combination with 10 mg vitamin E twice daily for six to twelve weeks. Vitamin E works to neutralize the bacteria in the sebum and, in the process, helps to reduce the inflammation of the acne lesions.

Success has also been reported in studies using zinc, although experts can't precisely pinpoint how the mineral undermines bacteria. Zinc helps regulate the function of the sebaceous oil glands and is known to play a role in many aspects of skin health and development. Research indicates that men and women with acne have lower zinc levels compared with people who do not have acne, and the more severe the acne, the lower the zinc levels. Studies have shown that people treated with zinc experience a greater reduction in acne inflammation when compared with those who given a placebo.

Various studies over the years have shown that high doses of vitamin A can be effective in controlling acne because skin cells depend largely upon the nutrient for their development. Vitamin A can also unclog skin pores and shrink oil glands if taken at high doses. Original research showing that vitamin A improved acne cases led to the development of a drug derived from this nutrient. The drug known as Accutane (isotretinoin) is sometimes prescribed to treat acne.

There is a problem in taking high doses of vitamin A and the drug Accutane, however. Their use can cause toxicity and serious side effects such as skin peeling and dryness; extensive damage to the liver; severe headaches from increased pressure within the head, or intracranial pressure; pain in the long bones; and profound birth defects if taken during pregnancy. Accutane can also cause depression, psychosis, and, rarely, suicidal tendencies.

My recommendation is not to use high doses of vitamin A exceeding 4,000 international units (IU), to treat acne, because of the frequent and severe side effects. Studies have shown that vitamin A taken in doses of 25,000 to 50,000 IU daily can control acne, but those sky-high doses will likely produce sometimes dangerous side effects. If you follow the other recommendations in this chapter regarding diet and supplementation, the chances are pretty good that you will not need to take high doses of vitamin A to combat acne.

While taking high-potency oil of oregano capsules and using the topical cream is often a successful strategy in clearing up acne, the best results are seen when these forms of the herbs are used in conjunction with the high-potency multivitamin and mineral formula, the essential oils, the detoxifying booster, and the digestive enzyme-prebiotic described earlier in the book. It's important to note that taking essential oils may increase the oily feel of the skin and actually aggravate some conditions. However, remember that essential oils promote anti-inflammatory hormones that help reduce the immune inflammatory response and improve the skin texture. My experience suggests that some acne patients may need to limit their intake of the essential oils supplement to one capsule a day, instead of two to three, as I usually recommend for healthy skin.

There is no doubt in my mind that proper nutrition and supplementation could alleviate at least part of the difficulties that teenagers and young adults face. (See Chapter 8 for a complete summary of how to treat acne.)

CURING ROSACEA

Rosacea is a chronic skin rash that appears on the nose and other parts of the face most often in fair-skinned middle-aged adults. It can also cause inflammation around the eyes. The condition has a harsh effect on many of the sebaceous glands, which become inflamed and infected in the areas where outbreaks occur.

For years, rosacea remained a mystery to the medical profession, and researchers could discover neither a cause nor a cure for the affliction. Now research indicates the rash seen in rosacea patients is often due to infection by a parasite called demodex, a mite known to infest the hair follicles and sebaceous ducts. Another study implicates a bacteria that infects the stomach lining and secretes a toxin that causes the inflammation and redness typical of rosacea. The condition disappears when antibiotics kill the bacteria.

Rosacea is known to be aggravated by the consumption of hot drinks, alcohol, and spicy foods. Other irritants include too much sun, extreme temperatures of either air or water, excessive physical activity, and stress. Rosacea can also be aggravated in women by an imbalance of estrogen and progesterone, which will be addressed in Chapter 7.

Oil of oregano has been proven effective in killing the mites that cause rosacea. Dr. Ingram's studies have shown that the high-potency form of oil of oregano is the most effective at killing the skin mite demodex to significantly improve the skin's condition in most instances. Recommended treatment for rosacea includes both oral supplements of the oil and topical applications.

1. Take one to two high-potency capsules twice daily.

2. Apply the topical cream directly to the infected areas each night before bedtime.

As support for oil of oregano in the treatment of rosacea, I recommend supplementation with the high-potency multiple vitamin and mineral formula, plus the essential oils, the detoxifying booster, and the combination of digestive enzymes and prebiotics. The most effective treatment for rosacea is a multifaceted nutrition and supplementation plan. Clearing impurities from the bloodstream with the immune detox booster and encouraging the growth of friendly bacteria by taking digestive enzymes and prebiotics is key in containing the immune inflammatory reactions that can aggravate rosacea and other skin conditions. (See Chapter 8 for specific details on how to treat rosacea.)

CURING FINGERNAIL AND TOENAIL FUNGUS

The incidence of fingernail and toenail fungus is increasing at an epidemic rate in North America. It's a serious, disfiguring condition that millions of people live with everyday.

Nail fungus has either one of two sources. It is most often produced by dermatophytes, organisms related to ringworm and athlete's foot. It can also be a product of a nasty little microbe called *Candida albicans.* The fungus settles deep into the nail bed and feasts off the rich nutrients in the skin cells. There it becomes quite comfortable, like a bad house guest that won't leave. And because the fungus is so far imbedded under the nail, topical remedies aren't powerful enough by themselves to penetrate deep down where it will be most effective.

Success Story
Miss SB Conquers Both Adult Acne and Rosacea

IN HER LATE THIRTIES, MISS SB developed a moderate case of adult acne that was compounded by the simultaneous development of rosacea. Never before in her life, even as an adolescent, had she experienced complexion problems of any kind. When she initially consulted her physician, he thought that her problem might be triggered by the type of birth control pill she had been using, and made an attempt to find an oral contraceptive that would help alleviate the problem. Despite her doctor's attempts to regulate estrogen and progesterone levels using various drugs, both the acne and the rosacea persisted.

Once the diagnosis of rosacea was confirmed in addition to acne, Miss SB's doctor prescribed an antibiotic to kill the skin mite that causes rosacea and to help reduce the acne bacteria at the same time. Aware of the possible side effects of taking antibiotics for prolonged periods, Miss SB came to me in search of an alternative method of treatment for her conditions. I explained the importance of taking vitamins, minerals, and essential oils to maintaining skin health, as well as boosting detoxification activity to clear the bloodstream of impurities that might be triggering immune inflammatory reactions and making her conditions worse. I started her on a high-potency multivitamin and mineral formula, plus essential oils and a detox booster, but her response to these supplements in the first two months was less than I had hoped. In response, I added two capsules twice daily of the high-potency oil of oregano supplement to her treatment program and instructed her to apply the oil of oregano topical lotion to her face at bedtime. Within two weeks of using the oil of oregano products, Miss SB's skin was 40 to 50 percent improved. Within four to six weeks there was an 80 to 90 percent improvement, with virtually no sign of rosacea. Her complexion had completely returned to normal with two months. Amazed and relieved to find a natural, safe, effective solution to her complexion problems, Miss SB told me that many of her friends had commented on her dramatic improvement and asked how she had achieved these results.

That was one of the first cases in which I incorporated oil of oregano into the treatment program for acne and rosacea. I was surprised myself to see not only how effective it was in treating those cases, but how quickly results became apparent with these very stubborn conditions.

Many factors increase the chances of developing nail fungus. These include excessive sugar intake, alcohol consumption, and poor hygiene. Chemical interaction with the skin—either through mild products like nail polish or through household detergents and stronger industrial products—increases the chances of developing nail fungus.

However, while reducing external opportunities to come in contact with the bacteria is helpful, the condition can develop from within just as easily, as the yeasts and fungi that cause the problem already exist within the body.

The best method of eradicating fingernail and toenail fungus is to use high-potency oil of oregano products, in both oral and topical forms. In addition to taking two capsules of oil of oregano twice a day to treat the fungal infection from the inside-out, you also need to rub the oil of oregano ointment twice daily on the nail bed and skin affected by the fungus. Soon you'll see significant improvements as these troublesome and stubborn fungal infections shrink or disappear.

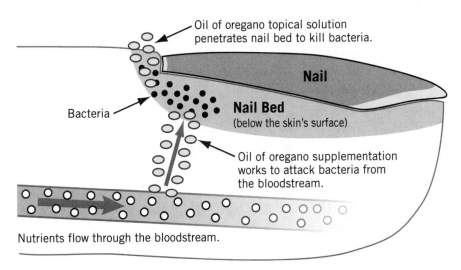

FIGURE 6.2. Oil of oregano works both topically and internally to eradicate fungus in the nail bed.

CURING PSORIASIS AND ECZEMA

In recent years, a number of scientific studies have shown that streptococci and *Staphylococcus aureus* bacteria are present in the skin lesions of people with psoriasis and eczema, where they promote inflammatory reactions that may aggravate these conditions. Numerous studies have shown that recurrent streptococcal infections can initiate psoriasis in children or aggravate existing psoriatic conditions. Emerging evidence suggests the combination of bacterial infections within the skin and bacterial toxins circulating in the bloodstream either initiates or aggravates certain cases of psoriasis and eczema.

In response to these discoveries, some practitioners and researchers have tested the use of antibiotics in treating psoriasis and eczema. Often, patients who are treated with antibiotics have seen a dramatic reduction in their number of skin lesions. However, the same researchers caution that while treatment with antibiotics can by helpful, long-term use of antibiotics can give rise to problems with multiresistant bacteria—new strains of bacteria that cannot be killed by antibiotics. They also point out that the majority of hospital-based infections in some countries are caused by these multiresistant bacteria.

This is where the work of Dr. Cass Ingram has proven to invaluable. He and fellow researchers have shown that high-potency oil of oregano effectively kills the bacteria that foster the development of psoriasis and eczema. In fact, as Dr. Ingram highlights in lectures and interviews, he has used oil of oregano successfully to manage his own psoriatic skin lesions. After reading his work and meeting him, I have chosen to include this form of oil of oregano in my supplementation plans for both psoriasis and eczema.

Treating Psoriasis and Eczema

As in the case of acne, high-potency oil of oregano can be used safely and successfully as a replacement for antibiotics in many cases of psoriasis and eczema. The supplement has demonstrated an amazing ability to kill off bacteria when taken orally in conjunction with topical application to the skin lesions. I now recommend using it as follows:

1. Take one to two high-potency capsules twice daily.

2. Apply the topical cream directly to the infected areas twice daily.

See Chapter 8 for the complete treatment plan.

CHAPTER 7

Female Hormonal Balance: How It Affects the Skin and Total Well-Being

We have seen throughout this book that optimal nutritional support is a must for skin cells to develop properly. However, women often must address another factor in order to achieve healthy-looking skin. Female hormones play an important role in determining the skin's appearance and texture, and to a significant degree, they affect a woman's overall feeling of well-being.

HORMONAL IMBALANCE SPELLS TROUBLE FOR YOUR SKIN AND REPRODUCTIVE ORGANS

Hormonal imbalance throws off the body's ability to function normally. Tissues that rely on these hormones are affected in ways that lead to a variety of female health complaints and problem skin conditions. This imbalance of reproductive hormones causes many women to experience acne breakouts in the days leading up to their periods. Studies clearly demonstrate that hormones such as estrogen, progesterone, and testosterone affect the texture and appearance of the skin, and an imbalance of these hormones results in complexion problems and aggravates skin disorders.

If your goal is to have clear, soft, healthy skin, it would be wise for you to understand the role hormones play in the overall picture of attaining and maintaining skin health. Unfortunately, hormonal imbalance is a widespread problem in younger women today due partly to improper nutrition and harmful lifestyle practices. As a result, a large percentage of younger women today suffer from various female health ailments.

The same underlying hormonal imbalances that promote poor health conditions also contribute to the bad complexion problems many of these women face, and they may aggravate other skin conditions as well. So it is vitally important for women not only to supply their bodies with the nutrients we discussed in the preceding chapters, but also to realize the importance of to improving complexion and skin texture and achieving an overall feeling of well-being.

Today, young women are suffering more and more from PMS, fibrocystic breast disease, uterine fibroids, and endometriosis, among other ailments. These conditions, along with a higher incidence of acne and other skin complexion problems, have been linked to hormonal imbalance in the estrogen-to-progesterone ratio—either estrogen blood levels are too high or progesterone blood levels are too low. Contributing to this imbalance may be poor dietary habits, such as eating too much animal fat and refined sugar and not enough fiber; impaired liver detoxification of circulating estrogens; and lack of exercise.

Hormonal imbalance can also affect skin in older women. During menopause, women experience a 90 percent drop in estrogen levels and a 66 percent drop in progesterone levels. This leads to "thinning" skin or skin atrophy, which affects the skin's appearance and texture.

Until recently, hormone replacement therapy had been the treatment of choice for many menopausal and postmenopausal women. However, with the discovery in 2002 that hormone replacement therapy increases the risk of breast cancer, heart attacks, and stroke, many women have become reluctant to use these drugs. Later in this chapter, we will look at natural hormone replacement strategies that have been shown to work in various clinical trials and that represent a safe alternative to medical hormone treatments.

YOUNGER WOMEN: HORMONAL IMBALANCE AND ITS EFFECT ON THE SKIN AND TOTAL WELL-BEING

Each month, many young women are burdened with recurring premenstrual syndrome, often referred to as PMS. Premenstrual syndrome brings on a number of physical and emotional symptoms that usually become noticeable seven to fourteen days before the start of the period and disappear when menstruation begins. PMS affects about one-third of all premenopausal women, mainly those twenty-five to forty years of age. About 10 percent of women affected by PMS suffer from a very severe form of the condition; their

Hormone Imbalance in Younger Women

Younger (menstruating) women can experience many unpleasant symptoms and conditions if their reproductive hormones are not balanced. Hormone imbalance in younger women can cause the following:

- Acne
- PMS
- Endometriosis

- Uterine fibroids
- Fibrocystic breast disease

symptoms are extreme and often include excruciating menstrual cramps and painful menstruation, or dysmenorrhea.

Common symptoms of PMS include mood swings, irritability, anxiety, fatigue, abdominal bloating, cramping, breast tenderness, headaches, backache, and swelling of fingers and possibly limbs, although not every woman experiences all the symptoms at one time. Many women also complain of a feeling of weight gain, increased aggressiveness, depressed mood, changes in libido, lethargy, food cravings, and skin disorders. PMS symptoms tend to fall into four main categories:

1. Behavioral: nervousness, anxiety, irritability, mood swings, fatigue, lethargy, depression.

2. Gastrointestinal: abdominal bloating, diarrhea and/or constipation, appetite changes with cravings for sugary or salty foods, or chocolate.

3. Reproductive tissue: breast tenderness and swelling, uterine cramping.

4. Other: headache, backache, acne, swelling in fingers or ankles, altered libido.

Many women who suffer from PMS experience acne breakouts or a change in skin quality at the same time their PMS symptoms show up. Because skin problems and PMS symptoms are related to hormonal imbalance, some doctors recommend the birth control pill for these women, so that the high levels of estrogen and progesterone in the pill will override the body's inability to balance these hormones naturally. However, there is a more natural way to balance and regulate hormone function, which I will describe below.

It should also be noted that higher circulating levels of testosterone and testosterone-related hormones called androgens are also associated with acne in women. That happens when the drop-off in estrogen and progesterone just prior to menstruation allows testosterone-related hormones to become more dominant in their effects on many tissues—including the skin—during the premenstrual and menstrual period. Testosterone-related hormones affect the skin by enlarging and stimulating the sebaceous oil glands to secrete excess sebum and keratin, which together can clog the openings of hair follicles. The bacteria that are found in the clogged follicles can, in turn, cause an infection that becomes apparent as an acne lesion. That explains why body builders and other athletes who take anabolic steroid drugs, which are androgens, often develop acne.

Hormone Imbalance and PMS

One of the main factors linked to PMS is an imbalance in the estrogen-to-progesterone ratio—high estrogen levels and low progesterone levels—five to ten days before a woman's period. This can happen because too much estrogen is being produced, not enough estrogen is being cleared out of the body due to poor liver detoxification, or not enough progesterone is being released by the corpus luteum, which forms in the ovaries after ovulation. If fertilization does occur, the corpus luteum shrinks and the release of progesterone drops off until about day fourteen of the next menstrual cycle, when a new corpus luteum forms in the ovaries after another ovulation. (The corpus luteum is the yellow sac that remains behind in the ovary after releasing the ripened egg [ovulation]. The corpus luteum is responsible for the majority of progesterone synthesized by a woman's body.)

Evidence shows a high-estrogen-to-low-progesterone ratio is also linked to a decline in brain endorphin levels. Brain endorphins are chemicals that make us feel good emotionally, so it makes sense that lower brain endorphin levels may contribute to mood swings as a symptom of PMS.

Increased estrogen levels are known to negatively affect levels of vitamin B_6, which are often low in depressed patients, especially women taking estrogens in the form of birth control pills or estrogen replacement therapy. At the same time, studies show that supplementing with vitamin B_6 can reduce many PMS symptoms.

Too much estrogen can also lead to increased levels of the hormone prolactin, which is associated with breast pain and fibrocystic breast disease.

Meanwhile, higher levels of aldosterone, which is the hormone that increases sodium and water retention, causes a feeling of bloating.

The imbalance in the estrogen-to-progesterone ratio explains, in part, why women experience many of the emotional and physical symptoms of PMS. Correcting this imbalance is key to relieving the symptoms of PMS and, at the same time, in improving skin texture and appearance.

Correcting the Estrogen-to-Progesterone Ratio Naturally

In many cases, PMS can be managed naturally with adjustments in the diet, some exercise, and the right nutritional supplements. These same nutrition, lifestyle, and supplementation strategies also provide relief to many women who suffer from fibrocystic breast disease, uterine fibroids, and endometriosis. That's because, like PMS, all these conditions are driven by estrogen. The nutrition, lifestyle, and supplementation strategies listed below can help remedy the estrogen-to-progesterone imbalance that contributes to these conditions and associated skin complexion problems.

1. Consuming a low-fat, high-fiber diet will help reduce levels of estrogen circulating in the blood. Studies reveal that when women lowered their fat intake from 40 percent to 25 percent of their total calories and increased their fiber consumption from 12 grams to 40 grams per day, there was a 36 percent reduction in blood estrogen levels. Women who are vegetarians take in higher amounts of fiber, and studies show they eliminate two to three times more estrogen from their bodies and have 50 percent lower levels of free estrogen in their blood than meat eaters. Fiber, especially wheat bran, binds to estrogen and drags it out of the body in bowel movements. Also thought to help this elimination are other sources of insoluble fiber, including flaxseed powder, psyllium husk fiber, corn and rice bran, beans, and peas.

2. Exercise has been proven to have a positive effect on reducing PMS frequency and severity. A number of studies show that women who follow a regular exercise program do not suffer from the frequent, severe PMS symptoms inactive women may tend to experience. In addition to lowering free-estrogen blood levels, exercise also raises brain endorphin levels, thereby improving mood and reducing anxiety and feelings of depression.

3. Specific dietary supplements are valuable in normalizing the estrogen-to-

progesterone ratio and noticeably lessening PMS frequency and severity. Black cohosh, soy isoflavones, B vitamins, and vitamin E are believed to be the most safe and effective.

Black Cohosh

Black cohosh (*cimifuga racemosa*) offers a safe, natural approach to the treatment of PMS and other reproductive tract disorders. It has no well-known drug-nutrient interactions and minimal side effects.

Research has shown that black cohosh contains the compounds triterpene and saponin, which act as natural building blocks from which the body can make more progesterone. Higher progesterone levels help balance the estrogen-to-progesterone ratio. At this time, black cohosh is the only known natural substance that can raise blood progesterone levels.

Physiologically, black cohosh extract appears to imitate the effects of estriol, which is a form of estrogen made by the body. Estriol is a weaker form of estrogen than other estrogens produced by the body, estrone or estradiol, and is not linked to increased risk of reproductive cancers. Like other forms of estrogen, estriol helps to maintain bone density and aids the body in removing cholesterol from the bloodstream. Black cohosh extract has also been shown to slow down the oversecretion of luteinizing hormone (LH), which is normally secreted by the pituitary gland when it senses that blood estrogen levels are low. This provides proof of the extract's estrogen-like properties.

Triterpenes in black cohosh help block the effects of excess estrogen on breast and uterine tissues. The active ingredients in black cohosh are known to have an antispasmodic effect on uterine tissues, reducing menstrual cramps. Black cohosh also acts as a natural anti-inflammatory and painkiller.

Studies of women with PMS reveal that the standardized grade of black cohosh can relieve PMS symptoms when taken at a dosage of 80 milligrams (mg), standardized to 2.5 percent triterpene content, once or twice daily. However, I feel that it is best to take black cohosh in a combination capsule that also contains 250 mg soy extract, standardized to 10 percent isoflavone content. Black cohosh and soy isoflavones work together to counteract the exaggerated effects of estrogen and boost progesterone production, helping to balance and better regulate the impact of these two hormones on reproductive and other tissues, including the skin. Because black cohosh and soy isoflavones work to balance estrogen and progesterone, the two herbal products may also block testosterone and other androgen hormones from over-stimulating the production of sebum and keratin from the sebaceous glands in the skin during the final days of the menstrual cycle, when estrogen and progesterone levels are normally very low. This helps to reduce acne break-outs; in fact, it is essentially the same manner in which birth control pills act to clear acne. However, while the two herbal substances have a similar action to birth control pills, they are not powerful enough to produce a contraceptive effect.

Soy Isoflavones

Like the active ingredients in black cohosh, soy isoflavones have been shown to counter the effects of the body's estrogens. When a woman's reproductive tissues are overstimulated by estrogen, hyperproliferation occurs, causing cells to divide and grow at a very rapid rate. Hyperproliferation is linked to increased risk of breast, endometrial, and cervical cancers, and it aggravates conditions such as fibrocystic breast disease, uterine fibroids, and endometriosis.

The active ingredients in soy extract—the isoflavones genistein and daidzein—produce a weak estrogenlike effect and slow down the rate of cell division. Soy isoflavones are phytoestrogens, or weak plant-based estrogens, that can attach to estrogen receptors on cells in the breast, endometrium, and other tissues. They compete with the stronger estrogen produced by the body, and therefore partially block the body's own estrogens from entering these tissues. This helps to reduce estrogen overstimulation in the breasts and the uterus.

Together as a team, black cohosh and soy isoflavones work to balance out the effects of estrogen and progesterone on female reproductive tissues. This relieves PMS symptoms, fibrocystic breast disease, and some cases of uterine fibroids and endometriosis. Both natural substances have also been shown to slow down the rate of cellular division in the breasts, decreasing the risk of breast cancer.

Soy isoflavones also improve estrogen detoxification by the liver and decrease estrogen production. All these functions help to regulate the normal estrogen-to-progesterone ratio, lessening the occurrence and severity of many female health conditions.

A landmark study published in a 2003 issue of *The Journal of Nutrition* showed that genistein, one of the isoflavones found in soy extract, helps to slow skin aging and significantly reduces cancerous changes to skin cells induced by sunlight. Genistein was shown to act in a manner similar to other antioxidants that protect skin cells from ultraviolet light and provide important biological anti-aging and anticancer effects in these cells. Soy isoflavones can also reverse skin dryness and vaginal dryness, and reduce the growth of facial hair in postmenopausal women. These findings strongly suggest that soy isoflavones exert their weak estrogenic effects on skin cells, which means that supplementation with soy isoflavones can favorably affect skin health, texture, and complexion. In my experience with clients and patients, that appears to be especially true when women take black cohosh and soy isoflavones together, because they act synergistically to reduce many female health complaints and improve skin health.

B Vitamins

More than a dozen studies suggest that vitamin B_6 supplementation is useful in treating PMS. Vitamin B_6 is a cofactor in estrogen detoxification in the liver, in the production of mood elevating brain chemicals called neurotransmitters, and in the formation of anti-inflammatory prostaglandin hormones. In some of these applications, vitamin B_6 works together with other B vitamins, such as niacin, folic acid, and vitamins B_2 and B_{12}. It's best to take a complete B-50 complex, which includes all the B vitamins as part of a high-potency multivitamin and mineral supplement, when treating PMS and related conditions.

Some studies suggest that vitamin B_6 should be taken in combination with 300 to 400 mg magnesium daily because the vitamin and mineral work together in many enzyme systems that lessen PMS symptoms. This also supports supplementation with a high-potency multivitamin and mineral formula.

Vitamin E

Studies suggest that supplementing with 400 international units (IU) a day of vitamin E can reduce various symptoms of PMS, including nervous tension, headache, fatigue, depression, insomnia, breast tenderness, anxiety, and food cravings. Vitamin E is known to modulate the production of prostaglandin hormones and directly affects cellular maturation and the rate of cell division in breast and other reproductive tissues. Supplementing vitamin E with 400 to 600 IU daily has also been shown to help regulate hormones in relation to PMS and fibrocystic breast disease.

In Chapter 1 you learned that taking 400 IU daily of vitamin E stimulates enzymes that increase the conversion rate of the essential oils GLA and EPA into the prostaglandin hormones PG-1 and PG-3, which make skin softer, smoother, moister, and more radiant. The same effect has been shown in regard to cells in breast tissue. Vitamin E aids in the conversion of GLA and EPA into PG-1 and PG-3 in breast cells, where the prostaglandins reduce inflammation and help alleviate breast tenderness associated with PMS and fibrocystic breast disease. PG-3 also slows the rate of cellular division in breast tissue, an effect that is linked to a decreased risk of breast cancer. The Nurses' Health Study, which followed 83,234 registered female nurses in the United States, reported that, after controlling for other risk factors, women in the top 20 percent of those taking vitamin E showed a 16 percent lower risk of breast cancer than women in the bottom 20 percent, after controlling for other risk factors. More recently, in a twelve- to fourteen-year follow-up study of vitamin E supplementation in breast cancer survivors, showed that women who took vitamin E had a 25 to 35 percent reduction in breast cancer recurrence, compared with women who did not take vitamin E, after controlling for other nutrition and lifestyle factors. Experimental studies of vitamin E have demonstrated that it has numerous anticancer effects, in addition to its role as an antioxidant and its ability to promote PG-3 synthesis.

Additionally, studies show that vitamin E supplementation not only reduces sun damage to the skin and improves skin texture in conjunction with essential oil supplementation, but also has important implications in preventing and managing various female health conditions. Having weighed all of this evidence, I feel strongly that women should take a daily supplement of 400 IU vitamin E in its all-natural form, d-alpha-tocopherol succinate.

The Hormone-Balancing Plan to Help You Feel Your Best and Improve Your Complexion

Struggles with unbalanced hormone levels can be a thing of the past. I have seen many women who suffer from PMS regain control of their hormone levels and improve their general feeling of well-being. They have also seen improvement in their complexions by following the recommendations listed here. The following dietary and lifestyle modifications should be adopted when dealing with fibrocystic breast disease, uterine fibroids, and endometriosis:

1. Reduce the amount of animal fat in your diet.

2. Consume more grain fiber in the form of wheat bran and flaxseed powder, and cruciferous vegetables, including cabbage, cauliflower, broccoli, Brussels sprouts, and bok choy. Cruciferous vegetables increase estrogen detoxification in the liver, and the indole-3-carbinol constituents in these foods act as phytoestrogens, helping to reduce the effects of the body's more powerful estrogens on female reproductive tissues.

3. Take a high-potency multivitamin and mineral supplement containing a B-50 complex, 400 IU vitamin E from natural sources, 200 mg magnesium, 500 mg calcium, and all nutrients from vitamin A to zinc as detailed in Chapter 2.

4. Take a female hormonal support product daily that contains 80 mg black cohosh, standardized to 2.5 percent triterpene content, and 250 mg soy extract, standardized to 10 percent isoflavones, and yielding 25 mg of isoflavones. This supplement should also contain 150 mg gamma-oryzanol to help balance testosterone function. (See Resources.)

5. Supplement your diet with soy-based foods, including soy milk and cheese, veggie burgers, miso, and tofu.

6. Take a detoxifying booster supplement to speed up the elimination of excess estrogen from the bloodstream. The supplement should include the recommended dosages of milk thistle, indole-3-carbinol, astragalus, and reishi mushroom extract outlined in Chapter 4.

7. Try an aerobic-based exercise program three to six times a week for twenty to forty-five minutes per session. Aerobic exercise increases blood flow through the liver, enabling liver cells to more efficiently remove excess estrogen from the circulation. Aerobic exercise also increases blood levels of sex-hormone-binding globulin (SHBG), which binds to estrogen in the bloodstream, reducing the ability of estrogen to bind to estrogen receptors on breast and other reproductive tissues. As such, elevated SHBG blood levels help to tone down the effects of estrogen on reproductive tissues. The rise in SHBG is a result of the reduction in insulin secretion that occurs with aerobic exercise and improved physical fitness. When insulin levels go down, it triggers increased synthesis and release of SHBG by the liver.

8. In cases where abdominal pain and cramping are recurring PMS symp-

toms, it's a good precaution to have a chiropractor examine your lower spine and pelvis. Nerve reflexes to and from the uterus and spine can increase painful menstruation problems. Chiropractic therapy has been shown to interrupt this cycle by reducing spinal nerve pressure or abnormal nerve reflexes that travel back and forth between the lower back and the uterus.

For a summary of nutrition and supplementation recommendations for PMS, fibrocystic breast disease, uterine fibroids, and endometriosis, see Chapter 8.

Success Story
Miss JA Puts Painful Menstruation and PMS Behind Her

Miss JA was a forty-year-old woman who had suffered as a teenager and again since her late thirties from excruciating menstrual pain in her lower abdomen, extending laterally to the area around both ovaries. The first two days of her menstrual period were so painful she had to stay in bed, and though she fought to endure the pain as best she could, she was often forced to take frequent doses of acetaminophen in order to bear the pain. She also gained five pounds during the premenstrual period due to excess swelling and bloating related to water retention, which made her feel sluggish and overweight.

During my consultation with Miss JA, I discussed the effectiveness of black cohosh and soy isoflavones in managing PMS symptoms and explained that black cohosh extract contained active antispasmodic ingredients that reduce painful menstruation in a number of clinical studies. Miss JA began taking the woman's hormonal balance product, which contains black cohosh, soy isoflavones, and gamma-oryzanol, which may help to block the exaggerated effects of testosterone in younger women. Five months later, she told me that the supplement had completely alleviated the pain of menstruation. "My periods now sneak up on me, and I don't even know that I am premenstrual," she said. "There is no weight gain or bloating, and I have absolutely no menstrual pain in my abdomen at all any more."

This is a remarkable story, but it's not uncommon. Other practitioners have seen similarly dramatic improvement after patients who suffer from menstrual cramping, uterine fibroids, and endometriosis began taking the appropriate supplements.

OLDER WOMEN: HORMONAL IMBALANCE DURING AND AFTER MENOPAUSE AND HOW IT AFFECTS THE SKIN AND TOTAL WELL-BEING

Menopause represents a challenging stage of a woman's life. During the menopausal years, most women experience a significant decline in hormone levels: a 90 percent decrease in estrogen and a 66 percent decrease in progesterone. The sudden decline in hormones triggers a number of menopausal signs and symptoms such as hot flashes, profuse sweating, mood disturbances, headaches, and accelerated aging of the skin, hair, and reproductive tissues. Additionally, if the proper precautions are not taken, calcium may be leached from the bones, leading to an increased risk of fractures.

When it comes to skin health and appearance, the drop-off in estrogen levels results in a decrease in collagen synthesis within the dermis, usually beginning after the age of forty. That accounts for much of the skin atrophy that occurs in subsequent years. Women using estrogen replacement have seen a reversal, or at least a minimizing, of skin atrophy because of estrogen's positive effects on collagen synthesis in the skin. Unfortunately, as we've already discussed, hormone replacement therapy (HRT) has been shown to increase the risk of breast cancer, heart attack, and stroke. The good news is there are some safe, natural substances that have an action similar to that of estrogen, and they can help prevent skin aging, atrophy, and dryness. These beneficial substances are known as selective estrogen receptor modulators, or SERMs for short. Some SERMs are synthetic drugs, but the SERMs

---

Hormone Imbalance in Older Women

Perimenopausal, menopausal, and postmenopausal women may experience a host of symptoms and illnesses when they no longer produce reproductive hormones as they once did. Hormone imbalance in older women can cause the following:

- Hot flashes
- Profuse sweating
- Mood disturbances
- Headaches
- Accelerated aging of the skin, hair, and reproductive tissues
- Increased risk of osteoporoctic fractures

that hold the greatest promise are those that come from natural sources, such as soy isoflavones and black cohosh extract. A groundbreaking study, published in a 2003 issue of the *International Journal of Molecular Medicine,* showed that a SERM called raloxifene, which has an estrogenlike action, can attach to estrogen receptors in skin cells and stimulate collagen synthesis—in some cases doing a better job than estrogen itself.

Research has also demonstrated that the soy isoflavone genistein and the active ingredients in black cohosh also mimic estrogen and prevent atrophy and dryness of vaginal tissues in postmenopausal women. Studies show that in addition to reducing hot flashes and related menopausal symptoms, supplements containing soy isoflavones and black cohosh extract also help to reduce skin aging, atrophy, and dryness. Overall, the body of evidence indicates that soy isoflavones and black cohosh are safe and effective alternatives to hormone replacement therapy for the management of menopausal symptoms and general well-being, and that they provide significant anti-aging support for the skin.

The Problem with Hormone Replacement Therapy

Beginning in the 1970s, hormone replacement therapy (HRT) had become an increasingly common treatment for menopausal symptoms. Although HRT can improve some symptoms and help to prevent weak, brittle bones of osteoporosis, it also had risks. On July 9, 2002, researchers announced that they were stopping the American Women's Health Initiative (WHI) trial of 16,000 women taking HRT. The results showed that after 5.2 years, there was a 26 percent increased risk of breast cancer in the women using hormone replacement than in women taking the placebo.

Previous data from the Nurses' Health Study showed that for each year a woman remained on HRT, her risk of developing breast cancer increased by 2.3 percent. Therefore, a postmenopausal woman taking HRT for ten years had a 23 percent increased risk of developing breast cancer, compared with women who did not use HRT. After twenty years of hormone replacement therapy, a woman's risk of developing breast cancer was 46 percent greater than for a woman who never used HRT.

Bad news regarding ERT, or estrogen replacement therapy, which does not include progesterone, appeared in the July 17, 2002, issue of *The Journal of the American Medical Association.* In a follow-up study of 44,241 participants in the Breast Cancer Detection Demonstration Project, researchers discovered that ERT increased the risk of ovarian cancer, with a relative risk of 1.8 in women who used ERT for ten to nineteen years and a 3.2 relative risk in women using ERT for twenty or more years.

The Women's Health Initiative study also revealed that women taking HRT had a 41 percent increased risk of stroke and a 29 percent increased risk of heart attack, compared with women taking the placebo. Before these findings became public, many doctors promoted HRT as a way to reduce the risk of heart disease in postmenopausal women; however, the results of the WHI trial provided convincing evidence to the contrary.

As a result of these studies, which were widely reported by the popular media, a growing number of women are giving up HRT medication. Medical doctors have been instructed not to prescribe HRT for patients unless it is absolutely necessary and are instead advised to find alternative methods that are safer but as effective in treating menopausal symptoms and preventing osteoporosis. Today, most women are seeking more natural methods of managing menopausal signs and symptoms and preventing osteoporosis. And women who are on HRT are looking for ways to help reduce the known risks.

Herbs Hold the Answer

In North America today, women live one-third of their lives during the post-menopausal years. Helping women to improve their health and quality of life during these years should be the goal of any nutrition, supplementation, or lifestyle recommendations.

As a natural alternative to hormone replacement therapy, I recommend the supplement containing black cohosh, soy extract, and gamma-oryzanol described below. These three natural products have a proven ability to reduce menopausal symptoms, maintain sexual function, support bone health, and even lower cholesterol levels. (See Resources.)

Black Cohosh

Black cohosh standardized to 2.5 percent triterpene glycoside content is the most thoroughly studied and commonly used natural supplement for the management of menopausal symptoms. Since 1956, over 1.5 million menopausal women in Germany have used black cohosh extract with noted success and no significant side effects. The natural triterpene compounds produce a mild estrogenlike effect, making it helpful in maintaining the normal integrity and secretions of the vaginal lining and supporting its sexual function.

In studies of menopausal women taking black cohosh, the herb has been tested in head-to-head trials against hormone replacement therapy and anti-anxiety medications. In each case, black cohosh was as effective as—and in some cases, more effective than—prescription medications in:

- Reducing hot flashes.

- Reducing anxiety and depression.

- Reducing sweating and night sweats.

- Reducing insomnia.

- Maintaining the vaginal lining and its secretions.

- Improving overall feeling of well-being.

Success Story
Miss JT Stops Suffering from Moderate to Severe Perimenopausal Symptoms

MISS JT WAS IN HER MID-FORTIES and in the earliest stages of menopause (perimenopausal) when she began to experience some early menopausal symptoms. By age forty-five, she was significantly bothered by hot flashes, sweating, and bouts of insomnia—symptoms that many women usually experience in their early fifties. Miss JT was reluctant to take hormone replacement therapy to alleviate her symptoms because of the increased risk of breast cancer and other health problems associated with treatment.

During my consultation with Miss JT, I explained how black cohosh, soy isoflavones, and gamma-oryzanol work synergistically to combat menopausal symptoms, and I gave her literature that reviewed the human trials showing that these natural herbs safely and successfully control the discomforts of menopause. Within the first month of taking two capsules daily of the women's supplement, Miss JT reported that her hot flashes and other menopausal symptoms were reduced by more than 70 percent. After a year, her symptoms were significantly reduced. Miss JT continues to be grateful that she can rely on an all-natural herbal supplement to keep her feeling well through this very challenging period of her life.

Four major clinical trials involving black cohosh extract have shown that it successfully reduces discomforts of menopause, including hot flashes, profuse sweating, headaches, dizziness, nervousness and irritability, sleep disturbances, and mood changes.

The first study was conducted by 131 doctors, who together recruited 629 participants. Eighty percent of the patients experienced a reduction in physical and psychological symptoms associated with menopause within six to eight weeks of treatment with black cohosh extract. Significant improvement was noted in the following symptoms:

- Hot flashes
- Profuse sweating
- Headache
- Vertigo
- Heart palpitations

- Tinnitus (ringing in the ear)
- Nervousness and irritability
- Sleep disturbances
- Depressive moods

Only 7 percent of participants in this study reported mild, temporary stomach complaints.

A second study of black cohosh compared the herb's effects to those of ERT or valium for twelve weeks. Black cohosh outperformed both. The third study compared the effects of black cohosh with those of ERT or a placebo over twelve weeks. Black cohosh produced better results in controlling menopausal symptoms and greater improvement in the health of the vaginal lining than either estrogen or the placebo. Of the women in the group taking black cohosh, the number of daily hot flashes dropped from an average of five to less than one. In the estrogen group, this number dropped on average from five to three and a half hot flashes a day.

Finally, in the fourth study, black cohosh was compared with a placebo in a study of 110 women. The women in the group taking black cohosh showed significant reduction in menopausal symptoms and improved blood hormone measurements. In addition to relieving hot flashes, black cohosh once again produced impressive age-reversal results in the vaginal lining, as confirmed by vaginal smear analysis.

To use black cohosh in the treatment of menopausal symptoms, I recommend taking 80 mg, standardized at 2.5 percent triterpene glycoside content, taken twice daily. The herb is best taken as part of a combination product that also contains soy isoflavones and gamma-oryzanol, which work synergistically with black cohosh to give the best results.

Soy Isoflavones

Studies of soy isoflavone supplementation have produced some positive results in the treatment of menopausal symptoms. Classified as phytoestrogens, or plant estrogens, soy isoflavones are beneficial because they exert mild estrogenlike effects when the body's natural estrogen hormones decline after menopause.

A minimum of 50 mg soy isoflavones a day has been shown to reduce hot flashes and reverse vaginal dryness in postmenopausal women. Some studies of women taking soy isoflavone products show up to a 40 percent reduction in hot flashes. In addition to reducing a range of menopausal symptoms, another benefit of taking soy is that it keeps cholesterol levels within a safe range by lowering blood cholesterol levels 9 to 12 percent—an important factor in preventing heart disease.

Soy isoflavones may also provide a number of other protective effects, including antioxidant action against free radicals, slowing the rate of cellular division to reduce cancer risk, reducing production of the estrone hormone by slowing down the estrogen synthase (aromatase) enzyme in fat tissue, detoxifying potentially harmful chemicals and hormones, and competing with the body's own powerful estrogen for attachment on breast and other tissues. Soy isoflavones have also been shown to support bone mineral density in postmenopausal women.

Gamma-oryzanol

Gamma-oryzanol is a natural substance derived from rice bran oil that is used in Japan as a prescription medication for the treatment of hot flashes. The product also lowers cholesterol and triglyceride levels 8 to 12 percent, helping to reduce the risk of heart disease.

Supplementation with 150 mg gamma-oryzanol twice daily has been shown to reduce the release of luteinizing hormone (LH). Menopausal symptoms such as hot flashes, profuse sweating, and mood changes result indirectly from the oversecretion of LH, which happens naturally to kick off another ovulatory cycle.

In North America, gamma-oryzanol is a natural health product, not a pre-

---

Success Story
Miss MM Controls Menopausal Symptoms Naturally

Miss MM was a fifty-six-year-old woman who entered menopause in her early 50s and had since suffered through the physical and emotional roller coaster ride of hot flashes, night sweats, disturbed sleep, and feelings of anxiety. A believer in natural medicine who was skeptical about the safety of certain prescription drugs, Miss MM was reluctant to try hormone replacement therapy to help control her menopausal symptoms.

After a friend told her that she had benefited from taking an herbal supplement with black cohosh, soy isoflavones, and gamma-oryzanol to control menopausal symptoms, Miss MM became a willing candidate to try it. Within the first month, her hot flashes were significantly reduced in frequency and severity. She reported a dramatic reduction in night sweats, improved sleep with less restlessness, and reduced anxiety. Her life had become manageable again and the quality of her life and her feeling of well-being were greatly improved. During the next three consecutive months, her symptoms were significantly reduced.

This is a typical case. I have seen many other women report similar results during the past five or six years that I have recommended this herbal combination. Reports from other health practitioners confirm the same results for their perimenopausal and postmenopausal patients.

---

scription drug, and clinical studies show that it is a worthy addition to the alternative treatment for menopause. Clinical trials reveal that 67 to 85 percent of women treated with gamma-oryzanol experience a significant reduction in menopausal symptoms.

What's Not Good for You

Other herbal agents in the marketplace have been shown to help manage female health problems and menopausal symptoms, but virtually all of them are associated with significant and sometimes dangerous side effects. For instance, red clover isoflavones and angelica species (dong quai) can increase the risk of a bleeding disorder and of severe sun-induced dermatitis. With prolonged use, licorice root frequently causes high blood pressure.

Using scientific studies and my own clinical experience as a guide, I formulated a combination product containing the correct dosages and standardized grades of black cohosh, soy isoflavones, and gamma-oryzanol described earlier in this chapter. This type of natural hormone replacement not only reduces menopausal symptoms, supports bone density, and helps reduce the risk of heart attacks and stroke, but it also provides natural hormonal support to skin cells to combat accelerated aging of the skin, hair, and nails that begins in the menopausal years.

THE IMPORTANCE OF BALANCING HORMONES

We've addressed many issues in this chapter that deal with balancing estrogen and progesterone hormones as they relate directly or secondarily to the skin's appearance and the health challenges faced by young and older women alike. Perimenopausal, menopausal, and postmenopausal women all need to follow health-promoting nutrition practices and, where appropriate, include dietary supplements to help regulate hormones. This will automatically lead to healthier and better looking skin and an improved overall sense of well-being.

CHAPTER 8

Putting It All Together: The Essential Nutrition and Supplementation Program for All Skin Conditions

Now it's finally time to put all the pieces together. Let's take a look at the daily nutrition and supplementation skin-care program you should follow based on your specific and unique needs.

GENERAL STRATEGIES FOR HEALTHY SKIN

There are some strategies that make sense for everyone, regardless of skin type or various skin conditions. Following the recommendations listed below will help you achieve soft, smooth, radiant, and healthy skin, no matter what your situation.

- Reduce the buildup of AA and PG-2 in your skin cells by reducing your intake of high-fat meat and dairy products and by substituting olive, canola, and peanut oils for other vegetable oils.

- Supplement your diet with a combination of borage, flaxseed, and fish oils—30 percent EPA and 20 percent DHA—to increase the production of the prostaglandin hormones PG-1 and PG-3 within your skin cells.

- Nourish your skin cells each day with the antioxidants and B vitamins required to promote the PG-1 and PG-3 production; reduce free-radical damage that causes skin aging, wrinkles, and cancer; and help boost detoxification activity. In addition to consuming at least five servings daily of fruits and vegetables, you should also take a high-potency multivitamin and mineral supplement.

- After age twenty, apply an ultrapure encapsulated form of concentrated

HA serum topically to your face each morning and evening. HA holds moisture in the skin, preventing and reversing fine lines, crow's feet, and wrinkles.

- Drink at least six to eight 8-ounce glasses of filtered, spring, or distilled water each day to keep your skin hydrated from the inside-out.

GENERAL STRATEGIES FOR PROBLEM COMPLEXIONS AND VARIOUS SKIN CONDITIONS

People with complexion problems and various skin conditions need to take some extra steps to help clear impurities from the bloodstream or kill the bacteria, mites, or fungi that might be causing trouble. In addition to the recommendations we just discussed, if you have a complexion problem, acne, eczema, psoriasis, rosacea, seborrhea, or any other skin inflammatory condition, you need to include the following nutrition and supplementation strategies in your skin-care program:

- Boost your body's detoxification activity by consuming cruciferous vegetables—broccoli, Brussels sprouts, cabbage, cauliflower, and bok choy—and soy-based foods daily. For virtually all skin conditions, I recommend the use of a dietary supplement that contains milk thistle, indole-3-carbinol, astragalus, and reishi mushroom extract.

- Supplement your diet with a product that contains high-potency, full-spectrum digestive enzymes and the prebiotics FOS and inulin. This will help prevent toxins produced by unfriendly gut bacteria from entering the bloodstream and causing immune inflammatory reactions that cause or aggravate skin conditions and complexion problems.

- Cleanse the bowel of toxins by eating plenty of grain fiber from wheat, rice, and corn bran, or by taking 2 to 3 teaspoons a day of psyllium husk fiber or 2 tablespoons of flaxseed powder.

- If you suffer from acne, rosacea, psoriasis, eczema, or chronic fungal infections, use high-potency oil of oregano in both the topical and supplemental forms.

That's the general scheme of things, but let's take a look at the exact nutrition and supplementation recommendations that address specific skin problems or conditions you may be experiencing.

Normal, Fairly Healthy Skin

People who have fairly good skin to start with can achieve even healthier, more radiant skin by following the nutrition and supplementation practices described here. This program will also help you prevent skin aging, wrinkling, and cell mutations that can cause skin cancer.

Dietary and Lifestyle Considerations

1. AA encourages the production of PG-2, which prevents your skin from being as smooth and soft as possible. Reduce the buildup of AA within skin cells—and in all your body's cells, for that matter—by cutting down on the following foods:

   - High-fat meat and dairy products.

   - Corn, sunflower seed, safflower seed, and mixed vegetable oils.

   - Alcohol and hydrogenated fats, including margarine, commercial peanut butter, and shortenings.

2. Replace the above foods with the following:

   - Chicken, turkey, fish, and Cornish hen.

   - 1-percent milk or yogurt and low-fat cheeses with less than 3 percent milk fat.

   - Olive, canola, or peanut oil for salad dressings and to sauté and stir-fry foods.

Important Supplements

- Omega-3 fats: Omega-3 fats provide the building blocks for prostaglandin hormones that reduce inflammation and slow the overactive replication of skin cells. The production of PG-1 and PG-3 hormones makes the skin smooth, soft, and moist. The "good" omega-3 fats also reduce the buildup of AA, which is normally converted to PG-2, a hormone that makes the skin dry, rough, and scaly. Omega-3s do this by blocking the enzyme that converts LA and GLA to AA. Examples of omega-3 fats of importance to skin health include EPA, found in fish and fish oils, and ALA, found primarily in flaxseed oil.

- Gamma-linolenic acid: GLA found in borage oil is a building block of PG-1, which improves the texture and radiance of the skin.

- B vitamins: A number of B vitamins—especially B_6 and niacin—are necessary cofactors that speed up enzymes important to the production of PG-1 and PG-3, which make the skin smooth, soft, and moist.

- Antioxidants: Vitamins C and E, selenium, and zinc are required to support the enzymes within skin cells and reproductive tissues that promote the formation of PG-1 and PG-3, which give the skin a more elegant feel and radiant appearance.

Recommended Supplements

- High-potency multivitamin and mineral formula.

- Essential oil supplement containing flaxseed, borage, and fish oils.

- Ultrapure encapsulated HA.

Poor Complexion, Dark Circles under Eyes, and Gray/Ashy Discoloration of the Skin

People who generally have a poor complexion, dark circles under their eyes, or a gray or ashy hue to their skin usually suffer from a combination of marginal vitamin and mineral deficiencies and high blood levels of impurities or allergens that trigger immune inflammatory reactions. Nutrition and supplementation intervention is needed to correct the underlying deficiency states and cleanse the blood of any impurities that adversely affect general health and complexion.

Dietary and Lifestyle Considerations

Review and follow the dietary and lifestyle recommendations under Normal, Fairly Healthy Skin, above. In addition, avoid foods to which you have a sensitivity or intolerance.

Important Supplements

Refer to the recommendations listed under Normal, Fairly Healthy Skin, above, and review the information regarding omega-3 fats, gamma-linolenic acid, B vitamins, and antioxidants. Also, note that the following supplements are useful in treating poor complexion:

- Gamma-linolenic acid: GLA is known to make the skin smooth, soft, and moist, and to reduce inflammatory skin conditions.

- B vitamins: Marginal deficiencies of B vitamins have been linked to poor complexion.

- Detoxifying nutrients: Milk thistle and indole-3-carbinol work in the liver to enhance detoxification and cleanse the blood of toxins that can aggravate skin complexion problems. The prebiotics FOS and inulin and digestive enzymes act in concert to clear toxins from the intestinal tract, regulate immune function, and prevent partially digested proteins from entering the bloodstream where they could induce immune inflammatory reactions that can cause or aggravate complexion problems.

Recommended Supplements

- High-potency multivitamin and mineral formula.

- Essential oil supplement containing flaxseed, borage, and fish oils.

- Detox-immune support supplement containing milk thistle, indole-3-carbinol, reishi mushroom extract, and astragalus.

- Digestive enzyme and prebiotic combination supplement.

- Ultrapure encapsulated HA.

Dry, Rough, or Gooseflesh Skin (Perifollicular Hyperkeratosis)

Dry, rough skin is usually the result of an essential fatty acid deficiency or insufficiency state. In some cases, it may progress to a type of "gooseflesh" condition known as perifollicular hyperkeratosis, which is characterized by dry, rough skin with small, dry, bumpy lesions, usually starts on the back and the sides of the arms, and can also affect the lower legs and back. Perifollicular hyperkeratosis can be an early sign of vitamin A deficiency. Many health practitioners fail to recognize these symptoms as a nutritional deficiency or insufficiency state and so do not suggest dietary modifications and the correct supplements to turn rough, dry skin into soft, smooth skin within just one to two months.

Dietary and Lifestyle Considerations

Review and follow the dietary and lifestyle recommendations under Normal, Fairly Healthy Skin, above.

Important Supplements

Refer to the recommendations listed under Normal, Fairly Healthy Skin, above, and review the information regarding omega-3 fats, gamma-linolenic acid, B vitamins, and antioxidants. Also, note that the following supplements are useful in treating dry, rough skin and perifollicular hyperkeratosis:

- Omega-3 Fats: Clinical trials have shown that supplementing with omega-3 fats from sources such as fish and fish oils and flaxseed oil can be effective in the treatment of dry, rough skin conditions and in some cases of perifollicular hyperkeratosis. Omega-3 fats are the building blocks for the prostaglandin hormones PG-1 and PG-3 hormones that make the skin smooth, soft, and moist.

- Gamma-linolenic acid: GLA has been shown to help cases of dry, rough skin and perifollicular hyperkeratosis because it's a building block for the production of PG-1, which is known to make the skin smooth, soft, and moist, and to reduce inflammatory skin conditions

Recommended Supplements

- High-potency multivitamin and mineral formula.

- Essential oil supplement containing flaxseed, borage, and fish oils.

- Ultrapure encapsulated HA.

Acne Vulgaris

Affecting 80 percent of the population between the ages of twelve and twenty-five, acne vulgaris is the most common skin condition in North America. Acne occurs when the sebaceous glands in the skin produce too much oil, or sebum, which clogs up the tiny openings of the hair follicles. Clogged pores cause pimples, whiteheads, and blackheads on the face, neck, shoulders, back, or chest.

Sebaceous glands are at their largest size in newborns, but they shrink during childhood. In adolescents entering puberty, whose hormone levels are on the rise, the sebaceous glands enlarge once again and being to secrete more oil. The increased production of sebum is the reason acne is so common among adolescents and teenagers. Bumps appear on the skin because the sebum clogs hair follicles. Inside these bumps, called comedones, bacteria and yeast go to work on the sebum, releasing free fatty acids that cause the comedones to become inflamed and sometimes rupture.

Sebum levels rise when testosterone is converted into dihydrotestosterone (DHT) in skin cells. DHT acts directly on sebaceous glands to increase their size and metabolic activity. That's one reason why teenage boys are more likely than girls to develop acne.

The causes of acne are very complex and involve many different systems and chemicals within the body. Hormones and enzymes interact with the immune system, but each individual's body reacts differently. While, the most severe forms of acne are most often seen in men, acne is generally more persistent in women, who tend to have flare-ups prior to monthly menstrual periods. Of note is the fact that low-grade, persistent acne is often found in professional women, perhaps due to the presence of chronic stress, which is known to increase the secretion of the adrenal androgens testosterone and androstenedione. These hormones increase the size and secretions of sebaceous glands, increasing vulnerability to acne.

Dietary and Lifestyle Considerations

Review and follow the dietary and lifestyle recommendations under Normal, Fairly Healthy Skin, on page 115. While there is much controversy over the impact that diet has on the development and severity of acne, some evidence shows that the dietary modifications listed below may be helpful in some cases. Keep in mind, however, that more scientific research is required to yield conclusive findings.

- Reduce your intake of refined sugars.

- Cut down the amounts of high-fat animal products and hydrogenated fats—including margarine, commercial peanut butter, and shortenings— in your diet.

- Avoid fried foods.

- Avoid heavily salted foods.

Important Supplements

Refer to the recommendations listed under Normal, Fairly Healthy Skin on page 115, and review the information regarding omega-3 fats, gamma-linolenic acid, B vitamins, and antioxidants. Also, note that the following supplements are useful in treating acne:

- Selenium: Some evidence suggests that supplementing with 200 micrograms (mcg) selenium daily can be helpful in clearing up acne.

- Zinc: Clinical trials show that daily zinc supplementation at doses as low as 30 milligrams (mg) can be a beneficial acne treatment.

- Vitamin E: There is evidence that vitamin E may neutralize bacteria present in the sebum to reduce inflammation in acne lesions.

- Chromium: It appears that chromium helps regulate blood sugar levels by working synergistically with insulin, and may therefore help to reduce the severity of acne.

- Indole-3-carbinol: This phytonutrient derived from cruciferous vegetables is known to enhance the body's detoxification system, indirectly helping to clear the bloodstream of impurities that may aggravate acne.

- Milk thistle: The flavonoid content of milk thistle, known as silymarin, enhances overall liver detoxification, boosts liver glutathione levels, and repairs some existing damage to liver cells. Milk thistle has been used successfully to help treat a variety of skin conditions, including acne.

- Gugulipid: The guggulsterones in gugulipid (a yellowish gumlike resin derived from the Mukul myrrh tree) are known to help clear triglycerides (the form in which fat travels through the bloodstream and is stored in fat cells) and cholesterol from the bloodstream. One study showed that gugulipid supplementation outperformed tetracycline (a standard acne treatment) in a study of 90 acne patients, making it a promising component in the management of acne.

- Prebiotics: Prebiotics such as FOS and inulin encourage the growth and reproduction of friendly bacteria in the large intestine that promote good health. Friendly bacteria such as *Lactobacillus acidophilus* and *bifidus* are known to help cleanse the digestive tract of toxins, regulate immune function, and reduce hypersensitivity reactions that can affect the skin.

- High-potency, full-spectrum digestive enzyme: Because the absorption into the bloodstream of incompletely digested proteins and other foreign compounds is known to cause immune inflammatory reactions that affect skin conditions, taking a digestive enzyme with each meal may be helpful to ensure the complete breakdown of all food.

- Oil of oregano: The volatile oils in high-potency oil of oregano products have been shown to kill the bacteria that cause acne, thereby helping to control the condition. For best results, take a high-potency oral supplement twice daily and apply the topical night cream before bedtime.

- Vitamin A: Skin cells require vitamin A for normal growth and development. Many studies show that vitamin A supplementation can reverse acne to a significant degree. However, because toxicity can cause birth defects in the offspring of pregnant women taking high doses of the vitamin, supplementation with more than 5,000 international units (IU) a day must be prescribed and monitored by an attending physician.

Recommended Supplements

Many people experience improvement by following the nutrition and supplementation recommendations outlined here. However, cases of acne that have a strong genetic component may not always respond fully to nutrition and supplementation, so it is impossible to predict the degree to which one person will benefit over another.

- High-potency multivitamin and mineral formula.

- Essential oil supplement containing flaxseed, borage, and fish oils.

- Detox-immune support supplement containing milk thistle, indole-3-carbinol, reishi mushroom extract, and astragalus.

- Digestive enzyme and prebiotic combination supplement.

- Two high-potency oil of oregano capsules taken twice daily.

- High-potency oil of oregano topical cream applied daily at bedtime.

Add in More Severe Cases

- Extra zinc: 15 mg daily.

- Gugulipid: 500 mg standardized to 5 percent guggulsterone content three times daily (optional).

- Vitamin A: 25,000 to 50,000 IU daily. Note that this high dose of vitamin A should not be taken for more than three consecutive months at a time because of the risk of toxicity, which includes early symptoms such as skin peeling and dryness. High dosages of vitamin A increase the risk of birth defects in the offspring of women who become pregnant while taking more than 5,000 IU a day. These dosages should not be taken by anyone with liver disease. Consult your physician if you are considering taking the high levels of vitamin A recommended above.

Eczema (Atopic Dermatitis)

Dermatitis literally means "inflamed skin." The term encompasses a number of conditions that have symptoms of red, itchy skin. Eczema is a form of dermatitis that may appear as a dry, scaly rash or weepy, oozing blisters. Chronic eczema causes dry, red, flaky patches on the skin, most frequently on the face, neck, scalp, arms, elbows, wrists, and knees. The condition may be classified as one of two types. Contact dermatitis, or contact eczema, occurs when an irritating substance such as a chemical, cosmetic, wool, lanolin, or rubber shoes comes in contact with the skin. Nickel in jewelry is a common cause. Poison ivy also causes a form of contact eczema.

Atopic eczema is usually caused by inhaled or ingested allergens, such as foods, pollen, dust, or animal dander. Some experts contend that intestinal dysbiosis can promote atopic eczema. In dysbiosis, there is a disruption of the normal bacterial flora of the gut with a disproportionately high concentration of unfriendly bacteria. Therefore, supplementation that increases friendly gut bacteria can be helpful in reducing symptoms of eczema. Recent studies also show that eczema lesions contain various bacterial strains, such as streptococci or *Staphylococcus aureus,* which may aggravate this condition in some people. Additionally, these bacteria secrete toxins that circulate in the bloodstream and can contribute to the development of eczema or worsen the condition.

There are four main objectives in treating eczema: reducing inflammation, relieving itching, moisturizing dry patches, and killing the bacteria that have been shown to worsen this condition in certain cases. Appropriate dietary and supplementation strategies can help relieve some of these symptoms of eczema.

Dietary and Lifestyle Considerations

Review and follow the dietary and lifestyle recommendations under Normal, Fairly Healthy Skin on page 115. In addition, avoid environmental irritants and any foods to which you have a sensitivity or allergy.

Important Supplements

Refer to the recommendations listed under Normal, Fairly Healthy Skin on page 115, and review the information regarding omega-3 fats, gamma-linolenic acid, B vitamins, and antioxidants. Also, include the following supplements, detoxification nutrients, and immune regulators in your treatment program:

- Milk thistle and indole-3-carbinol: Milk thistle and indole-3-carbinol work in the liver to enhance detoxification and cleanse the blood of toxins and various allergens that can aggravate eczema.

- Prebiotics and digestive enzymes: Prebiotics, such as FOS and inulin, and digestive enzymes act in concert to rid toxins from the intestinal tract, regulate immune function, and prevent partially digested proteins from entering the bloodstream where they could induce immune inflammatory reactions that aggravate eczema. Prebiotics, which are food sources of friendly bacteria, help to increase the concentrations of friendly gut bacteria by prompting them to proliferate rapidly, crowding out unfriendly bacteria.

- Oil of oregano: High-potency oil of oregano has been shown in experimental studies to kill the bacteria that aggravate eczema. Anecdotal evidence suggests that some people with eczema benefit from taking a high-potency oil of oregano oral supplement, and applying a topical oil of oregano lotion on eczema lesions.

- Hyaluronic acid (HA): Topical application of HA may help heal eczema lesions, although the mechanism that produces these results is yet to be determined. I have seen this work in several cases of eczema, and I strongly recommend that people with eczema apply a topical HA serum to their lesions twice daily as an integral part of the global management of this condition.

Recommended Supplements

Many people experience improvement by following the nutrition and supplementation recommendations outlined here. However, cases of eczema that have a strong genetic component may not always respond to nutrition and supplementation, so it is impossible to predict the degree to which one person will benefit over another.

- High-potency multivitamin and mineral formula.

- Essential oil supplement containing flaxseed, borage, and fish oils.

- Detox-immune support supplement containing milk thistle, indole-3 carbinol, reishi mushroom extract, and astragalus.

- Digestive enzyme and prebiotic combination supplement.

- Ultrapure encapsulated HA, applied topically to eczema lesions twice daily, in addition to facial application.

- Two high-potency oil of oregano capsules taken twice daily.

- High-potency oil of oregano topical cream applied twice daily to eczema lesions.

Psoriasis

Approximately 2 percent of the American population has psoriasis, which is equally common in men and women and affects all age groups. Psoriasis is a chronic skin condition that causes cells to develop too rapidly, producing thick white or red patches on the knees, elbows, scalp, hands, feet, or lower back. Normally, skin cells mature gradually, with new cells continuously replacing those in the outer layers as they are shed or sloughed off about every twenty-eight days. In psoriasis, skin cells do not mature fully before they move to the surface quickly over three to six days. The cells build up on the surface, forming the characteristic red skin rash loosely covered with silvery white scales.

Some doctors believe that the immune system is a factor in the development of psoriasis because an increased number of white blood cells are present between the abnormal layers of skin. Studies have also shown that psoriasis responds to drugs that suppress the immune system.

An underlying factor that appears to contribute to the development of psoriasis is a high level of AA within skin cells. Remember, AA is converted into PG-2, a prostaglandin hormone that encourages inflammation and rapid cell division. Dietary and supplementation strategies aimed at decreasing AA buildup in skin cells have demonstrated impressive results in a number of clinical trials with psoriasis patients. Recent research shows that various bacterial strains, such as streptococci and *Staphylococcus aureus,* are found in psoriasis skin lesions, where they may aggravate the condition in some people. Additionally, these bacteria secrete toxins that circulate in the bloodstream and can contribute to the development of psoriasis or worsen the condition.

Warm weather and sunlight tend to improve psoriasis, while cold weather and stress tend to aggravate it. Psoriasis is sometimes associated with a serious joint arthritic condition known as psoriatic arthritis, which typically affects the hands, knees, wrists, elbows, and ankles.

Dietary and Lifestyle Considerations

Review and follow the dietary and lifestyle recommendations under Normal, Fairly Healthy Skin on page 115. In addition, eat more fiber-rich cereals and grains to clear toxins from the intestinal tract.

Important Supplements

Refer to the recommendations listed under Normal, Fairly Healthy Skin on page 115, and review the information regarding omega-3 fats, gamma-linolenic acid, B vitamins, and antioxidants. In addition, include the following supplements in your treatment program:

- Omega-3 fats: Clinical trials have shown that omega-3 fat supplementation is effective in treating psoriasis. Omega-3 fats give rise to PG-3, which helps slow down the replication of cells. PG-3 also reduces some of the inflammatory aspects of psoriatic skin lesions.

- Gamma-linolenic acid: GLA found in borage oil is a building block of PG-1, which is known to reduce inflammatory conditions of the skin.

- B vitamins: A number of B vitamins—especially B_6 and niacin—are necessary cofactors that speed up enzymes important to the production of anti-inflammatory prostaglandins in the skin.

- Antioxidants: Vitamins C and E, selenium, and zinc are required to support the enzymes within skin cells that promote the formation of prostaglandins known to slow the growth rate of skin cells and reduce inflammation.

- Detoxifying nutrients: Milk thistle and indole-3-carbinol work in the liver to enhance detoxification and cleanse the blood of toxins that aggravate skin conditions. The prebiotics FOS and inulin and digestive enzymes act in concert to clear toxins from the intestinal tract, regulate immune function, and prevent partially digested proteins from entering the bloodstream where they could induce immune inflammatory reactions that cause or aggravate skin conditions.

- Oil of oregano: High-potency oil of oregano has been shown in experimental studies to kill the bacteria that can cause psoriasis. Anecdotal evidence suggests that some people with psoriasis benefit from taking a high-potency oil of oregano oral supplement and applying topical oil of oregano lotion on psoriasis lesions.

Recommended Supplements

Many people experience improvement by following the nutrition and supplementation recommendations outlined here. However, cases of psoriasis that have a strong genetic component may not always respond fully to nutrition and supplementation, so it is impossible to predict the degree to which one person will benefit over another.

- High-potency multivitamin and mineral formula.

- Essential oil supplement containing flaxseed, borage, and fish oils.

- Detox-immune support supplement containing milk thistle, indole-3-carbinol, reishi mushroom extract, and astragalus.

- Digestive enzyme and prebiotic combination supplement.

- One to two high-potency oil of oregano capsules taken twice daily.

- High-potency oil of oregano topical cream applied twice daily.

Add in More Severe Cases

- Milk thistle: 200 mg daily (standardized to 80 percent silymarin content).

- Chromium: 300 mcg daily.

- Selenium: 100 mcg daily.

- Zinc: 15 mg daily.

- Psyllium husk fiber: 2 to 3 teaspoons daily; or flaxseed powder: 2 tablespoons daily.

Rosacea (Acne Rosacea)

Rosacea is a chronic skin condition of the forehead, cheeks, nose, and chin that occurs most often in adults ranging from thirty to fifty years of age, who have fair skin. The condition is more common in women than in men, at a ratio of about 3 to 1. Usually, the skin on or around the nose is red and swollen, with acnelike blemishes. The condition may progress to cause inflammation around the eyes, and the nose may become swollen.

There is still some debate about the cause of rosacea, but evidence suggests that the condition may be triggered or aggravated by factors including excess alcohol consumption, menopausal flushing related to hormonal imbalance, local infection from the skin mite demodex folliculorum, B-vitamin deficiencies, and intestinal tract disorders, such as digestive enzyme insufficiency.

Dietary and Lifestyle Considerations

Review and follow the dietary and lifestyle recommendations under Normal, Fairly Healthy Skin on page 115. In addition the dietary modifications listed below may be helpful in some cases:

- Eat more fiber-rich cereals and grains to clear toxins from the intestinal tract.

- Reduce your intake of coffee, alcohol, hot beverages, spicy foods, and any other food or drink that causes a flush.

Important Supplements

Refer to the recommendations listed under Normal, Fairly Healthy Skin on page 115, and review the information regarding omega-3 fats, gamma-linolenic acid, B vitamins, and antioxidants. In addition, include the following supplements in your treatment program:

- Oil of oregano: The volatile oils in high-potency oil of oregano products have been shown to kill the skin mite demodex folliculorum, which may cause rosacea, thereby helping to control the condition. Clinical evidence reveals that taking a high-potency oral supplement daily and applying a topical cream at night is helpful in these cases.

- Omega-3 fats: Clinical trials have shown that omega-3 fat supplementation is effective in reducing skin inflammatory conditions. Omega-3 fats give rise to PG-3, which reduces inflammation, slows the replication of cells, and blocks the conversion of linoleic acid to arachidonic acid, thereby reducing PG-2 levels.

- Gamma-linolenic acid: GLA found in borage oil is a building block of PG-1, which is known to reduce inflammatory conditions of the skin.

- B vitamins: Supplementation with B vitamins has been effective in treating rosacea. Vitamin B_2 (riboflavin) is possibly the most effective in these cases. Many B vitamins stimulate enzymes that are involved in the synthesis of PG-1 and PG-3, both of which reduce inflammation.

- Antioxidants: Vitamins C and E, selenium, and zinc are also required to support the enzymes within skin cells that promote the formation of prostaglandins known to slow the growth rate of skin cells and reduce inflammation.

- Detoxifying nutrients: Milk thistle and indole-3-carbinol work in the liver to enhance detoxification and cleanse the blood of toxins that aggravate skin conditions. The prebiotics FOS and inulin and digestive enzymes act in concert to clear toxins from the intestinal tract, regulate immune function, and prevent partially digested proteins from entering the bloodstream where they could induce immune inflammatory reactions that cause or aggravate skin conditions. Some studies show that patients with rosacea benefit from supplementation with a full-spectrum, high-potency digestive enzyme.

Recommended Supplements

Many people experience improvement by following the nutrition and supplementation recommendations outlined here. However, cases of psoriasis that have a strong genetic component may not always respond fully to nutrition and supplementation, so it is impossible to predict the degree to which one person will benefit over another.

- High-potency multivitamin and mineral formula.

- Essential oil supplement containing flaxseed, borage, and fish oils.

- Detox-immune support supplement containing milk thistle, indole-3-carbinol, reishi mushroom extract, and astragalus.

- Digestive enzyme and prebiotic combination supplement.

- Two high-potency oil of oregano capsules taken twice daily.

- High-potency oil of oregano topical cream applied daily at bedtime.

- Menopausal women who experience hot flashes that may aggravate rosacea should also take women's hormonal balance formula containing black cohosh, soy isoflavones, and gamma-oryzanol.

Seborrheic Dermatitis (Seborrhea)

Seborrheic dermatitis is a common inflammatory skin condition that, in mild cases, is characterized by a dry, flaky scalp, sometimes confused with severe dandruff. In more severe cases, symptoms may also include itching and burning, with greasy scales overlying red patches on the scalp. The condition can also affect other areas of the skin, including the forehead, eyebrows, eyelids, ears, armpits, chest, groin, and the skin folds beneath the breasts and between the buttocks. Nasolabial seborrhea occurs where the nose meets the face. Strong evidence shows that nutrition and supplementation are highly useful in managing this condition.

Although infants may develop seborrheic dermatitis—known in these cases as cradle cap—the following recommendations apply only to the adult condition.

Dietary and Lifestyle Considerations

Review and follow the dietary and lifestyle recommendations under Normal, Fairly Healthy Skin on page 115. In addition, avoid environmental irritants and any foods to which you have a sensitivity or allergy.

Important Supplements

Refer to the recommendations listed under Normal, Fairly Healthy Skin on page 115, and review the information regarding omega-3 fats, gamma-linolenic acid, B vitamins, and antioxidants. In addition, include the following supplements in your treatment program:

- Omega-3 fats: Clinical trials have shown that omega-3 fats are effective in dealing with inflammatory skin conditions. Omega-3 fats give rise to PG-3, which reduces inflammation, slows the replication of skin cells, and blocks the conversion of linoleic acid to arachidonic acid, thereby reducing PG-2.

- Gamma-linolenic acid: GLA found in borage oil is a building block of PG-1, which is known to be helpful in combating inflammatory skin conditions.

- B vitamins: Supplementation with a high-potency B complex has been shown to improve cases of seborrheic dermatitis. Skin cells require various B vitamins for their normal development and appearance, as well as to stimulate the enzymes that produce PG-1 and PG-3, both of which reduce inflammation of skin-related conditions.

- Antioxidants: Vitamins C and E, selenium, and zinc are also required to support the enzymes within skin cells that promote the formation of prostaglandins known to reduce skin inflammatory conditions.

- Detoxification nutrients and immune regulators: Milk thistle and indole-3-carbinol work in the liver to enhance detoxification and cleanse the blood of toxins and various allergens that aggravate inflammatory skin conditions. The prebiotics FOS and inulin and digestive enzymes act in concert to clear toxins from the intestinal tract, regulate immune function, and prevent partially digested proteins from entering the bloodstream where they may induce immune inflammatory reactions that cause or aggravate inflammatory skin conditions. Prebiotics, which are food sources of friendly bacteria, help to increase the concentrations of friendly gut bacteria by prompting them to proliferate rapidly, crowding out unfriendly bacteria.

Recommended Supplements

Many people experience improvement by following the nutrition and supplementation recommendations outlined here. However, cases of seborrheic dermatitis that have a strong genetic component may not always respond fully to nutrition and supplementation, so it is impossible to predict the degree to which one person will benefit over another.

- High-potency multivitamin and mineral formula.

- Essential oil supplement containing flaxseed, borage, and fish oils.

- Detox-immune support supplement containing milk thistle, indole-3-carbinol, reishi mushroom extract, and astragalus.

- Digestive enzyme and prebiotic combination supplement.

Add in More Severe Cases

Folic acid: 5 to 10 mg daily. Note that this is a very high dosage of folic acid that should be taken only under the close supervision of a physician.

Younger Women's Health Issues: PMS, Fibrocystic Breast Disease, Uterine Fibroids, and Endometriosis

Conditions in younger women related to the reproductive system—such as PMS, fibrocystic breast disease, uterine fibroids, and endometriosis—are caused or aggravated by an imbalance in the estrogen-to-progesterone ratio, in which estrogen levels are high and progesterone levels are low. This hormonal imbalance can also contribute to complexion problems, which often accompany female health problems, it's important to treat the underlying hormonal imbalance, in addition to treating the skin directly.

Dietary and Lifestyle Considerations

Review and follow the dietary and lifestyle recommendations under Normal, Fairly Healthy Skin on page 115. In addition, include the following strategies in your treatment program:

- Reduce the buildup of arachidonic acid (AA) in your skin cells. AA encourages the production of PG-2, which can increase inflammation of reproductive tissues, thereby aggravating conditions related to women's health.

- Eat more dietary fiber from sources such as wheat bran, psyllium husk, and flaxseed powder. Consuming a low-fat, high-fiber diet will help reduce levels of estrogen circulating in the blood because fiber binds to estrogen and drags it out of the body.

- Eat at least one serving daily of a cruciferous vegetable, such as broccoli, Brussels sprouts, cabbage, cauliflower, or bok choy. Cruciferous vegetables contain indole-3-carbinol, which speeds up estrogen detoxification in the liver. The same substance also acts as a plant-based estrogen, reducing the effects of the body's own powerful estrogens on the reproductive tissues.

Important Supplements

Refer to the recommendations listed under Normal, Fairly Healthy Skin on page 115, and review the information regarding omega-3 fats, gamma-linolenic acid, B vitamins, and antioxidants. In addition, include the following supplements in your treatment program:

- Omega-3 fats: Omega-3 fats provide the building blocks for prostaglandin hormones that reduce inflammation of the skin and reproductive tissues, as well as and other tissues. These "good" fats promote the development of PG-3, which acts as a natural anti-inflammatory to help relieve the symptoms of PMS, fibrocystic breast disease, uterine fibroids, and endometriosis.

- Gamma-linolenic acid: GLA found in borage oil is a building block for the production of PG-1, which reduces inflammatory conditions of the skin and other tissues.

- B vitamins: A number of B vitamins—especially B_6 and niacin—are necessary cofactors that speed up enzymes important to the production of PG-1 and PG-3. These prostaglandin hormones act as natural anti-inflammatory agents that reduce the swelling and pain accompanying PMS and other female reproductive problems. B vitamin supplementation has been used with great success in cases of PMS. Given that fibrocystic breast disease, uterine fibroids, and endometriosis also involve inflammatory processes, supplementing with B vitamins should be part of the management of these women's health problems.

- Antioxidants: Vitamin E supplementation has been used successfully to treat fibrocystic breast disease and to manage PMS.

- Detoxifying nutrients: Milk thistle and indole-3-carbinol work in the liver to enhance detoxification and cleanse the blood of toxins and excess estrogen that aggravate skin complexion problems and female reproductive conditions. The prebiotics FOS and inulin and digestive enzymes act in concert to clear toxins from the intestinal tract, regulate immune function, and prevent partially digested proteins from entering the bloodstream where they may induce immune inflammatory reactions that can cause or aggravate complexion problems and promote inflammatory reactions in other tissues.

Recommended Supplements

- High-potency multivitamin and mineral formula.
- Essential oil supplement containing flaxseed, borage, and fish oils.
- Detox-immune support supplement containing milk thistle, indole-3-carbinol, reishi mushroom extract, and astragalus.
- Digestive enzyme and prebiotic combination supplement.

- Female hormonal support supplement containing black cohosh and soy isoflavones. These substances are phytoestrogens, or plant-based estrogens, that compete with the body's own powerful estrogens, as well as those from the birth control pill and hormone replacement therapy. In this manner, phytoestrogens such as black cohosh and soy isoflavones reduce the effects of the more powerful estrogens on reproductive tissues. This has an important balancing effect on the estrogen-to-progesterone ratio and helps to alleviate many symptoms associated with PMS, fibrocystic breast disease, uterine fibroids, and endometriosis. The active ingredients in black cohosh also boost the production of progesterone, further helping to establish a healthier estrogen-to-progesterone ratio. Because hormonal balance is important to skin health and appearance, skin problems related to female conditions may improve with proper nutrition and supplementation.

- Flaxseed powder: Flaxseed powder contains plant-based estrogens, which block the action of the body's own powerful estrogens and prescription estrogens on reproductive tissues. The substance works synergistically with black cohosh and soy isoflavones to help balance the estrogen-to-progesterone ratio. For best results, take 2 tablespoons of flaxseed powder daily.

MENOPAUSAL AND POSTMENOPAUSAL WOMEN

During menopause, women experience a 90 percent decline in estrogen production and a 66 percent decline in progesterone production. The dramatic drop-off in these hormones triggers many degenerative changes in the early stages of menopause that can cause uncomfortable symptoms such as hot flashes, profuse sweating, insomnia, anxiety, and mood swings, to name a few. Hormonal changes also promote calcium loss from bone, increasing the risk of osteoporotic fractures, especially in the hip and spine. The decline in estrogen and progesterone allows the cells that line the vagina and other reproductive tissues to shrink up, or atrophy.

Skin is also affected by the dramatic drop in estrogen and progesterone levels. Without adequate hormonal support, the skin atrophies, becoming thinner and drier, less radiant, and more prone to wrinkles and general aging. A decrease in hair quality and luster and nail strength are also common complaints among postmenopausal women. The good news is that the proper nutrition and supplementation program can prevent and reverse many of these signs and symptoms, returning the body to a more youthful, vibrant level of functioning on both the inside and the outside.

Dietary and Lifestyle Considerations

Review and follow the dietary and lifestyle recommendations under Normal, Fairly Healthy Skin on page 115.

Important Supplements

Refer to the recommendations listed under Normal, Fairly Healthy Skin on page 115, and review the information regarding omega-3 fats, gamma-linolenic acid, B vitamins, and antioxidants. Also include omega-3 fats in your treatment plan. Omega-3 fats provide the building blocks for prostaglandin hormones that reduce inflammation of the skin and reproductive tissues, as well as other tissues.

Recommended Supplements

- High-potency multivitamin and mineral formula.

- Essential oil supplement containing flaxseed, borage, and fish oils.

- Female hormonal support supplement containing black cohosh, soy isoflavones, and gamma-oryzanol: This product provides the body with plant-based estrogens, which can compensate for the huge drop-off in estrogen that normally occurs during the menopausal years. The active ingredients in black cohosh and soy isoflavones are known to attach to estrogen receptors throughout the body, helping to slow the aging process by exerting moderate estrogenic effects on these tissues. Black cohosh has been shown to provide the same or better relief of menopausal symptoms as HRT in a number of clinical trials. Together, black cohosh and soy isoflavones maintain the structure and secretary function of the cells that line the vagina, and exert other anti-aging effects on skin cells throughout the body. Gamma-oryzanol, a highly effective natural ingredient derived from rice bran oil, is used in Asia as a prescription drug to treat hot flashes and related menopausal symptoms.

  For all these reasons, supplementing with a female hormonal support product has been shown to maintain bone density; improve the quality of the skin, hair, and nails; and promote a woman's overall feeling of well-being. Using black cohosh, soy isoflavones, and gamma-oryzanol represents a safer approach to the hormonal management of menopause than does the use of HRT, which has been shown to increase the risk of breast cancer, heart attack, and stroke.

- Calcium and vitamin D: In addition to the 500 mg calcium and the 400 IU vitamin D in the high-potency multivitamin and mineral supplement, post-menopausal women require extra supplementation with calcium and vitamin D to prevent osteoporosis. Based on the amount of calcium taken in from the diet, it's likely that menopausal women will require an additional 500 to 1,000 mg calcium to achieve a total daily calcium intake of 1,500 to 2,000 mg. And studies show that postmenopausal women who take 600 to 1,000 IU vitamin D from daily supplementation reduce the incidence of hip fractures on average by up to 50 percent.

- Flaxseed powder: Flaxseed powder contains plant-based estrogens that block the overproduction of dangerous estrogens linked to the increased risk of breast cancer in postmenopausal women. The plant-based estrogens in flaxseed powder from ground flaxseeds have also been reported to improve the texture of the skin. As an added benefit, the unique types of fiber in flaxseeds also prevent the development of gallbladder stones and congestion, common problems among postmenopausal women. For best results, 2 tablespoons of flaxseed daily should be included in any supplementation program to treat female health problems and related skin conditions.

Afterword

I hope you have enjoyed reading *The Wrinkle-Free Zone*. My goal has been to provide you with a concrete and scientifically based nutrition and supplementation plan to help you properly nourish your skin with the nutrients necessary to slow aging; create a smooth, soft, moist, clear, and radiant complexion; and treat existing skin conditions and complexion problems.

From my vantage point, with more than twenty years of helping patients, I assure you the information in this book is the missing link in skin-care management in our era. It is indeed time to appreciate the importance of balanced nutrition and supplementation to skin texture and appearance. Many nutrients may need to be taken at levels that exceed what a healthy diet alone can provide. This is why I recommend specifically targeted supplements for the skin, based on your skin types and any skin conditions you may have. Regardless of the quality of your skin today, or your skin quality over the years, you stand to benefit from taking the right nutritional supplements, as I have explained throughout *The Wrinkle-Free Zone*.

Fortunately, skin-care professionals across North America have started to embrace the use of nutrition and supplementation in the skin-care management of their patients and clients. This trend will undoubtedly continue as these professionals become more educated and trained about the science and clinical studies related to these interventions.

It is my hope that this book has given you the information you need to use specific and appropriate nutrition and supplementation strategies, as well as some natural topical treatments, including the topical use of HA, to enhance the health and appearance of your skin. And I hope that it will further stimu-late the interest in and use of nutrition and supplementation by the skin-care professional community.

I wish you the best of luck in your personal pursuit of a healthy complex-ion and overall wellness campaign. Eat smart, live well, take the supplements you need, and you'll look and feel great.

Resources

Over the years I have formulated a number of supplement products to meet the needs of my patients and have recommended these formulations to other heath-care practitioners. These formulations are presently under the Adëeva brand name and are fully explained on the Adëeva website at www.adeeva.com. As such, the Adëeva website makes specific reference to me as their product formulator and features many of the research papers and other educational materials I have developed, which explain the importance of nutrition and supplementation in skin-care management. Also note that while the Adëeva supplement products contain the exact formulations I recommend, there are other reputable manufacturers of nutritional supplements that you might be interested in investigating.

Dietary Supplements for Skin Support

I recommend the following to clients, skin-care professionals, and health practitioners:

- High-potency multivitamin and mineral supplement (brand name Adëeva Formula 1) contains the recommended levels of antioxidants, B vitamins, and other vitamins and minerals.

- Essential oils supplement (brand name Adëeva Formula 2) contains the recommended levels of flaxseed, borage, and fish oils.

- Detoxifying booster and immune system regulator (brand name Adëeva Formula 3) contains the recommended combination of milk thistle, indole-3-carbinol, reishi mushroom extract, and astragalus.

- Digestive enzyme and prebiotic supplement (brand name Adëeva Formula 4) contains the recommended full spectrum of digestive enzymes and the prebiotics FOS and inulin.

- Women's hormonal support supplement (brand name Adëeva Women's Hormonal Balance) contains the recommended dosages and standard grades of black cohosh, soy isoflavones, and gamma-oryzanol.

- High-potency oil of oregano ingestible capsules (brand name Adëeva Orega-Skin) contains the recommended dosage and potency of oil of oregano.

Topical Products for Skin Support

- Encapsulated hyaluronic acid (brand name Adëeva Essential H.A.) provides the recommended two-step system of spray mist and HA serum.

- Oil of oregano topical lotion (brand name Adëeva Oil of Oregano Topical Lotion) contains the recommended dosage of oil of oregano.

Where to Find Adëeva Products

Adëeva products are available at salons, spas, and skin-care clinics throughout North America. For a location near you, consult the store finder at the Adëeva website, www.adeeva.com, or call them at 1-888-494-1010.

Additional research on nutrition and skin-care management can be found at www.adeeva.com.

Other Topical Beauty Products

The following premier topical beauty products are available through esthetician salons, skin-care clinics, and spas:

- Moisturizer for oily skin: Guinot-Longue Vie Cellulaire; reduces oiliness of skin and helps to reduce breakouts, especially in T-zone area of the face.

- Anti-aging mask: Phytomer Ogénage; lifts, tightens, and firms the skin.

- Eye mask: Darphin Soothing Eye Contour Mask; soothes skin around eyes and reduces puffiness.

- Eye care: Oxygen Botanicals Eye Cream; apply overnight to help reduce fine lines.

- Cleanser and toner: YonKa cleanser and toner; a good cleanser and toner for all skin types.

- Body moisturizer: Oxygen Botanicals Super Hydrating Moisturizer for all skin types.

- Neck cream: Catherine Atzen The Neck Cream.

References

Chapter 1

Danno, K., Ikai, K., Imamura, S., "Anti-inflammatory effects of eicosapentaenoic acid on experimental skin inflammation models," *Arch Dermtol Res,* 285(7) (1993): 432–435.

Fishcher, S.M., "Is cyclooxygenase-2 important in skin carcinogenesis?" *J Environ Pathol Toxicol Oncol,* 21(2) (2002):183–191.

Horrobin, D.F., "Essential fatty acid metabolism and its modification in atopic eczema," *Am J Clin Nutr,* 71(1 Suppl) (January 2000): 367S–72S.

Manku, M.S., Horrobin, D.F., Morse, N., et al, "Prostaglandins," *Leukot Med,* 9(6) (December 1982): 615–628.

Miller, C.C., Tang, W., Ziboh, V.A., Fletcher, M.P., "Dietary supplementation with ethyl ester concentrates of fish oil (n-3) and borage oil (n-6) polyunsaturated fatty acids induces epidermal generation of local putative anti-inflammatory metabolites," *J Invest Dermatol,* 86(1) (January 1991): 96–103.

Murray, M., Pizzorno, J., *Encyclopedia of Natural Medicine* (revised 2nd edition), Prima Publishing 1998: 448–454.

Murray, M., *The Encyclopedia of Nutritional Supplements,* Prima Publishing, 1996: 249–278.

Pustisek, N., Lipozencic, J., "Prostaglandins in dermatology," *ADC (Acta Dermatovenerol Croat),* 9(4) (December 2001): 291–298.

Raederstorff, D., Loechleiter, V., Moser, U., "Polyunsaturated fatty acid metabolism of human skin fibroblasts during cellular aging," *Int J Vitam Nutr Res,* 65(1) (1995): 51–55.

Reichert, R., "Evening primrose oil cream, dry skin, and atopic disposition," *Quarterly Review of Natural Medicine,* (Spring 1998): 7

Ziboh, V.A., "Implications of dietary oils and polyunsaturated fatty acids in the management of cutaneous disorders," *Arch Dermatoil,* 125(2) (February 1969): 241–245 EPA And Skin Health.

Ziboh, V.A., Miller, C.C., Cho, Y., "Metabolism of polyunsaturated fatty acids by skin epidermal enzymes: generation of anti-inflammatory and anti-proliferative metabolites," *Am J Clin Nutr,* 71(1 Suppl) (January 2000): 361S–6S

Chapter 2

Aesoph, L.M., "A holistic approach to skin protection," *Nutrition Science News,* 3(4) (1998): 204–208.

Boelsma, E., et al., "Nutritional skin care; health effects of micronutrients and fatty acids," *American Journal of Clinical Nutrition,* 73(5) (2001): 853–864.

Callens, A., et al., "Does hormonal skin aging exist? A study of the influence of different hormone therapy regimens on the skin of postmenopausal women using non-invasive measurement techniques," *Dermatology,* 193(4) (1996): 289–294.

Demetriou, A.A., et al., "Vitamin A and retinoic acid: induced fibroblast differentiation in vitro," *Surgery,* 98 (1985): 931–934.

Eberlein-Konig, B., et al., "Protective effect against sunburn of combined systemic ascorbic acid (vitamin C) and d-alpha-tocopherol (vitamin E)," *J Am Acad Dermatol,* 38(1) (1998): 45–48.

Emonet-Piccardi, N., et al., "Protective effects of antioxidants against UVA-induced DNA damage in human skin fibroblasts in culture," *Free Radic Res,* 29(4) (1998): 307–313.

[AUTHORS??] "Estrogen: Skin, Aging & Prevention." *Modern Medicine,* 65(5), (May 1997): 26.

Firkle, T., et al., "Antioxidants and protection of the skin against the effect of ultraviolet rays," *Cas Lek Cesk,* 139 (12) (2000): 358–60.

Gensler, H.L., et al., "Oral niacin prevents photocarcinogenesis and photoimmunosuppression in mice," *Nutr Cancer,* 34(1) (1999): 36–41.

Guttman, C., "Estrogen receptors: scalp physiology," *Dermatology Times,* 21(9) (September 2000): 42.

Halpern S., editor, *Clinical Nutrition* (2nd edition), J.B. Lippincott Company, (1987): 399–406.

Henderson, A., "Skin, aging and treatment," *Women's Health Weekly,* Issue N (October 7 1996–October 14 1996): 19.

Hendler, S., *The Doctors' Vitamin and Mineral Encyclopedia,* New York, Simon and Schuster, 1990: 195–207 (Zinc).

Hoffman, R.L., "The holistic MD: skin (part one): conscious choice," *The Journal of Ecology & Natural Living,* 15 (1991): 24.

Keller, K.L., Fenske, N.A., "Uses of vitamins A, C, and E and related compounds in dermatology: a review," *J Am Acad Dermatol,* 39(4 pt 1) (1998): 611–625.

Kragballe, K., "The future of vitamin D in dermatology," *J Am Acad Dermatol,* 37 (3 pt 2) (1997): S72–S76.

Krause, M. and Mahan, K. editors, *Food, Nutrition and Diet Therapy* (7th edition) W.B. Saunders Company (1984): 119–132.

Morimoto, S., et al., "An open study of vitamin D_3 treatment in psoriasis vulgaris," *Br J Dermatol,* 115 (1986): 421–429.

Nutrition for Living (2nd edition), The Benjamin/Cummings Publishing Companies, Inc., 1988: 12–14, 338.

Nutrition in Perspective (2nd edition), New Jersey, Prentice-Hall, Inc., 1987.

Pizzorno, J., "Normalizing inflammatory function," *Total Wellness,* Prima Publishing, 1996: 163–191.

Podda, M., et al., "UV irradiation depletes antioxidants and causes oxidative damage in a model of human skin," *Free Radic Biol Med,* 24(1) (1998): 55–65.

Pressman, A, and Adams, A., *Clinical Assessment of Nutritional Status: A Working Manual.* Management Enterprises, New York, 1982: 29–36

Pugliese, P.T., "The skin's antioxidant systems," *Dermatol Nurs,* 10(6) (1998): 401–416; quiz 417–418.

Reavley, N. editor, *The New Encyclopedia of Vitamins, Minerals, Supplements and Herbs,* (M. Evans and Company, Inc. 1998: 310–328 (Zinc): 668–676 (Skin Conditions).

Seifter, E., Crowley, L.V., et al., "Influence of vitamin A on wound healing in rats with femoral fracture," *Ann Surg,* 181 (1975): 836–841.

Shukla, A., "Depletion of reduced glutathione, ascorbic acid, vitamin E and antioxidant defense enzymes in a healing cutaneous wound," *Free Radic Res,* 26(2) (1997): 93–101.

Stahl, W., et al., "Carotenoids and carotenoids plus vitamin E protect against ultraviolet light-induced erythema in humans," *Am J Clin Nutr,* 71(3) (March 2000): 795–798.

United States Department of Agriculture, Food Technology, The National Health and Nutrition Examination Survey II (NHANES II) 35 (1981): 9.

Werbach, M., *Nutritional Influences on Illness,* California, Third Line Press, Inc., 1987.

Chapters 3 and 4

Akiyama, M., et al, "Arteriovenous haemangroma in chronic liver disease: clinical and histopathological features of four cases," *Br J Dermatol,* 144 (2001): 604–609.

Andrews, G., et al., "Seborrheic dermatitis: supplemental treatment with vitamin B_{12}," *NY State J Med,* (1950): 1921–1925.

Belew, P., et al., "Endotoxemia in psoriasis," *Arch Dermatol,* 118 (1982): 142–143.

Bittiner, S., et al., "A double-blind randomized placebo-controlled trial of fish oil in psoriasis," *Lancet,* 1 (1988): 378–380.

Burkitt, D., et al., "Effects of dietary fiber on stools and transit time and its role in the causation of disease," *Lancet,* 11 (1972): 1408–1412.

Callaghan, T., "The effect of folic acid on seborrheic dermatitis," *Cutis;* 3 (1967): 584–588.

Crotty, B., "Ulcerative colitis and xenbiotic metabolism," *Lancet,* 343 (1994): 35–38.

Hollander, D., et al., "Aging-associated increase in intestinal absorption of macromolecules," *Gerontology,* 31: 133–137

Isolauri, E., et al., "Probiotics: effects on immunity," *Am J Clin Nutr,* 73 (suppl) (2001): 444–450.

Madara, J., et al., "Structure and function of the intestinal epithelial barrier in health and disease," *Gastroenterol Pathol,* 9 (1990): 306–432.

Majarmaa, H., et al., "Probiotics: a novel approach in the management of food allergy," *J Allergy Clin Immunol,* 99 (1997): 179–186.

Michaelson, G., et al., "Erythrocyte glutathione peroxidase activity in acne vulgaris and the effect of selenium and vitamin E treatment," *Acta Derm Venerol,* 64 (1984): 9–14.

Murray, M., and Pizzorno, J., *Encyclopedia of Natural Medicine,* Prima Health, 1998: 104–125.

Nisenson, A., "Treatment of seborrheic dermatitis with biotin and vitamin B complex," *J Ped,* 81 (1972): 630–631.

Pizzorno, J., *Total Wellness,* Prima Publishing, 1996: 87–162.

Rosenberg, E., et al, "Microbiol factors in psoriasis," *Arch Dermatol,* 118 (1982): 1434–1444.

Savolainen, J., et al., "Candida albicans and atopic dermatitis," *Clin Exp Allergy,* 23 (1993): 332–339.

Schrezenmeir, J., et al., "Probiotics, prebiotics, and synbiotics – approaching a definition," *Am J Clin Nutr,* 73 (Suppl) (2001): 361–364.

Skinner, R., et al., "Improvement of psoriasis with cholestyramine," *Arch Dermatol,* 118 (1982): 144.

Snider, B., et al., "Pyridoxine therapy for premenstrual acne flare," *Arch Dermatol,* 110 (1974): 103–111.

Takagi, Y., et al., "Coexistence of psoriasis and linear IgA bullous dermatosis," *Br J Dermatol,* 142 (2001): 513–516.

Thurman, F., "The treatment of psoriasis with sarsparilla compound," *N Engl J Med,* 227 (1942): 128–133.

Wallace, J., "Pathogenesis of nonsteroidal anti-inflammatory drug gastropathy: recent advances," *Eur J Gastro Hepatol,* 5 (1093): 403–407.

Weber, G., et al, "The liver as a therapeutic target in dermatoses," *Med Weltz,* 34 (1983): 108–111.

Chapter 5

Agren, U.M., Tammi, R.H., Tammi, M.I., "Reactive oxygen species contribute to epidermal hyaluronan catabolism in human skin organ culture." *Free Radic Biol Med,* 23(7) (1997): 996–1001.

Brown, T.J., Alcorn, D., Fraser, J.R., "Absorption of hyaluronan applied to the surface of intact skin," *J Invest Derm,* 113(5) (1999): 740–746.

Encapsulated Hyaluronic Acid: Anti-wrinkle Agent. Cosmetic Manufacturers Inc.

Liguori, V., Guillemin, C., Pesce, G.F., et al., "Double-blind, randomized clinical study comparing hyaluronic acid cream to placebo in patients treated with radiotherapy," *Radiother Oncol,* 42(2) (1997): 155–161.

Pugliese, P., *Physiology of the Skin II,* Allured Publishing, 2001: 13–14.

Shepard, S., Becker, H., Hartmann, J.X., "Using hyaluronic acid to create a fetal-like environment in vitro," *Ann Plast Surg,* 36(1) (1996): 65–69.

Trabucchi, E., Pallotta, S., Morin, M., et al., "Low molecular weight hyaluronic acid prevents oxygen free-radical damage to granulation tissue during wound healing," *Int J Tissue React,* 24(2) (2002): 65–71.

Chapter 6

Alt HealthWatch, database Product Profiles: Oil of Oregano: Natural herbal supplement offers a variety of remedies, MMRC, *Health Educator Reports,* 2000.

Blumenthal, M., Busse, W.R., Goldberg, A., et al., (editors). *The Complete German Commission E Monographs: Therapeutic Guide to Herbal Medicines,* Boston, MA: Integrative Medicine Communications, 1998: 358–359.

Dorman, H.J., et al., "Antimicrobial agents from plants: antibacterial activity of plant volatile oils," *J Appl Microbiol,* 88(2) (February 2000): 308–316.

Force, M., Sparks, W.S., Ronzio, R.A., "Inhibition of enteric parasites by emulsified oil of oregano in vivo," *Phytotherapy Research: PTR,* 14(3) (May 2001): 213–214.

Hammer, K.A., Carson, C.F., Riley, T.V., "Antimicrobial activity of essential oils and other plant extracts," *J Appl Microbiol,* 86 (1999): 985–990.

Ingram, C., D.O., "The respiratory solution: wild oregano – the most potent germicide," *Consumer Health Newsletter,* 25(4), (April 2002): 6.

Ingram, C., D.O., "Wild Oregano: Germ Killing Spice," *MMRC Health Educator Reports,* (2000): 2.

Ingram, C., D.O., *The Cure Is in the Cupboard,* Knowledge House, 1997.

Komine, M., Tamaki, K., "An open trial of oral macrolide treatment for psoriasis vulgaris" *Journal of Dermatology,* 27(8) (August 2000): 508–512.

Leung, A.Y., Foster, S., *Encyclopedia of Common Natural Ingredients* (2nd edition), New York, John Wiley & Sons, 1996: 398–399.

Leung, D.Y., Hauk, P., Strickland, I., Travers, J.B., Norris, D.A., "The role of superantigens in human diseases: therapeutic implications for the treatment of skin diseases," *British Journal of Dermatology,* 139 (Suppl 53) (December 1998): 17–29.

Marino, M., Bersani, C., Comi, G., "Impedance measurements to study the antimicrobial of essential oils from Lamiaceae and Compositae," *International Journal of Food Microbiology,* 67(33) (August 5 2001): 187–195.

Noah, P.W., "The role of microorganisms in psoriasis," *Seminars in Dermatology,* 9(4) (December 1990): 269–276.

Paravina, M., Randjelovi, H., Risti, G., Tiodorovi, J., "Staphylococcus and skin diseases-incidence and antibiotic sensitivity," *Srpski Arhiv Za Celokupno Lekarstvo,* 117(5–6) (May–June 1989): 335–340.

Peirce, A., *Practical Guide to Natural Medicines,* New York: William Morrow and Co., 1999, 476–477.

Piquero-Casals, J., Fonseca de Mello, A.P., Dal Coleto, C., Fonseca Takahashi, M.D., Simonsen Nico, M. M., "Using oral tetracycline and topical betamethasone valerate to treat acrodermatitis continua of hallopeau," *Cutis; Cutaneous Medicine for the Practitioner,* 70(2) (August 2002): 106–108.

Ponce, M.M., Navarro, A.I., Martinez, G.M.N., et al., "In vitro effect against Giardia of 14 plant extracts," *Rev Invest Clin,* 46 (1994): 343–347 [in Spanish].

Rosenberg, E.W., Noah, P.W., Skinner, R.B., Jr., "Microorganisms and psoriasis," *Journal of the National Medical Association,* 86(4) (April 1994): 305–310.

Skinner, R.B., Jr., Rosenberg, E.W., Noah, P.W., "Antimicrobial treatment of psoriasis," *Dermatologic Clinics,* 13(4) (October 1995): 909–913.

Skov, L., Baadsgaard, O., "Bacterial superantigens and inflammatory skin diseases," *Clinical and Experimental Dermatology,* 25(1) (January 2000): 57–61.

Solntseva, V.K., Bykov, A.S., Vorob'ev, A.A., Ivanov, O.L, Solntsev, V.V., Bykov, S.A., "Skin microbiocenosis in patient with chronic deramatoses," *Zhurnal Microbiologii, Epidemiologii, I Immunobioligii,* 6 (November–December 2000): 51–55.

Stiles, J.C., Sparks, W., Ronzio, R.A.. "The inhibition of *candida albicans* by oregano," *J Applied Nutr,* 47 (1995): 96–102.

Tantaoui, E.A., Beraoud, L., "Inhibition of growth and aflatoxin production in *Aspergillus parasiticus* by essential oils of selected plant materials," *J Environ Pathol Toxicol Oncol,* 13 (1994): 67–72.

Thestrup-Pedersen, K., "Bacteria and the skin: clinical practice and therapy update," *British Journal of Dermatology,* 139 (Suppl 53) (December 1998): 1–3.

Tisserand, R., Balacs, T., *Essential Oil Safety,* New York, Churchill Livingston, 1996: 156–157.

Veien, N.K., "The clinician's choice of antibiotics in the treatment of bacterial skin infection," *British Journal of Dermatology,* 139 (Suppl 53) (December 1998): 30–36.

Wilson, J.K., Al-Suwaidan, S.N., Krowchuk, D., Feldman, S.R., "Treatment of psoriasis in children: is there a role for antibiotic therapy and tonsillectomy?" *Pediatric Dermatology,* 20(1) (January–February 2003): 11–15.

Chapter 7

"British scientists say HRT trial should continue," *Reuters Health Information,* 2002.

Kaunitz, AM, "Use of combination hormone replacement therapy in light of recent date from the Women's Health Initiative," *Medscape Women's Health Journal,* July 12, 2002.

Dawson-Hughes, B., "Calcium supplementation and bone loss: a review of controlled clinical trials," *American Journal of Clinical Nutrition,* 54 (1991): 274S–280S.

Nelson ME, Fiatarone, MA, Morganti CM, et al., "Effects of high-intensity strength training on multiple risk factors for osteoporotic fractures: a randomized controlled trial," *JAMA,* 272(4) (1994): 1909–1914.

"Health after 50," *John Hopkins Medical Newsletter,* 11(9) (November 6–7, 1999).

"Isoflavones and menopause," *Medical Post,* (October 3, 2000).

Henderson JW, Donatelle RJ, "Complementary and alternative medicine use by women after complete of allopathic treatment for breast cancer," *Alternative Therapies,* 10(1) 2004: 52–57.

"Optimal calcium intake: NIH Consensus Panel," *JAMA,* 272(24) (1994): 1942–1948.

Dawson-Hughes B, "Rates of bone loss in postmenopausal women randomly assigned to one of two dosages of vitamin D," *American Journal of Clinical Nutrition,* 61 (1995): 1140–1145.

Chapuy, MC, Arlot, ME, Duboeuf, F, et al. "Vitamin D_3 and Calcium to Prevent Hip Fractures in Elder Women," *New England Journal of Medicine,* 327 (1992): 1637–1642.

Abraham, G.E., "Nutritional factors in the etiology of the premenstrual tension syndrome," *J Reprod Med,* 28 (1983): 446–464.

Aganoff, J.A., et al., "Aerobic exercise, mood states and menstrual cycle symptoms," *J Psychosom Res,* 38 (1994): 183–192.

Albertzazzi, P., et al., "The effect of dietary soy supplementation on hot flashes," *Obstet Gynecol,* 91 (1998): 6–11.

Anderson, J.W., et al., "Meta-analysis of the effects of soy protein intake on serum lipids," *N Engl J Med,* 333 (1995): 276–282.

Barclay, L., M.D., "Estrogen therapy, but not estrogen-progestin: linked to ovarian cancer," *JAMA,* 288 (2002):334–341, 368–369.

Barnhart, K.T., et al., "A clinician's guide to the premenstrual syndrome," *Med Clin North Am,* 79 (1995): 1457–1472.

Bendich, A., "The potential for dietary supplements to reduce premenstrual syndrome (PMS) symptoms," *J Am Coll Nutr,* 19 (2000): 3–12.

Berman, M.K., et al., "Vitamin B_6 in premenstrual syndrome," *J Am Diet Assoc.* 90 (1990): 859–861.

Bermond, P., "Therapy of side effects of oral contraceptive agents with Vitamin B_6," *Acta Vitaminol-Enzymol,* 4 (1982): 45–54.

Bougnoux, P., Koscielny, S., Chajès, V., Descamps, P; Couet, C., Calais, G., "Alpha-linolenic acid content of adipose breast tissue: a host determinant of the risk of early metastasis in breast cancer," *British Journal of Cancer,* 70(2) (August 1994): 330–334.

Brinton, L.A., "Menopausal estrogen use and risk of breast cancer," *Cancer,* 47(10) (1981): 2517–2522.

Budieri, D., Li Wan, Po, A., Doman, J.C., "Is evening primrose oil of value in the treatment of premenstrual syndrome?" *Control Clin Trials,* 17 (1996): 60–68.

Cassidy, A., et al., "Biological effects of a diet of soy protein rich in isoflavones on the menstrual cycle of premenopausal women," *Am J Clin Nutr,* 60 (1994): 333–340.

Castelli, W.P., Griffin, G.C., "How to help patients cut down on saturated fat," *Postgraduate Medicine,* 84(3) (1988): 44–56.

Chiechi, L.M., Putignano, G., Guerra, V., Schiavelli, M.P., Cisternino, A.M., Carriero, C., "The effect of soy rich diet on the vaginal epithelium in post menopause; a randomized double blind trial," *Maturitas,* 45(4) (August 20, 2003): 241–246.

Choi, P.Y., et al., "Symptom changes across the menstrual cycle in competitive sportswomen, exercisers, and sedentary women," *Br J Clin Psychol,* 34 (1995): 447–460.

Chuong, C.J., et al., "Periovulatory beta-endorphin levels in premenstrual syndrome," *Obstet Gynecol,* 83 (1995): 755–760.

Colditz, G A., "Relationship between estrogen levels, use of hormone replacement therapy and breast cancer," *J Natl Cancer Inst,* 90(11) (1998): 814–823.

Colgan, M., *Hormonal Health,* Canada, Apple Publishing, 1996.

Collins, A., Cerin, A., Coleman, G., Landgrein, B.M., "Essential fatty acids in the treatment of premenstrual syndrome," *Obstet Gynecol,* 17 (1993): 60–68.

Connelly, D.M., "An acupuncturist looks at women's health," *Meridians,* 1(2) (June 1, 1993): 18–20.

Deadman, P., "Acupuncture in the treatment of premenstrual syndrome," *Journal of Chinese Medicine,* (May 1, 1995): 5–14.

Dittmar, R.W., et al., "Premenstrual syndrome, treatment with a phytopharmaceutical," *Therapiewache Gynakol,* 5 (1995): 60–68.

Dixon-Shanies, D., Shaikh, N., "Growth inhibition of human breast cancer cells by herbs and phytoestrogens," *Oncol Rep,* 6(6) (1999): 1383–1387.

Eriksson, E., "Serotonin reuptake inhibitors for the treatment of premenstrual dysphoria," *Int Clin Psychopharmacol,* 14 (Suppl 2) (May 1999): S27–S33.

Facchinetti, F., et al., "Oestradiol/Progesterone imbalance and the premenstrual syndrome," *Lancet,* 2 (1985): 1302.

Facchinetti, F., Sances, G., Borella, P., et al., "Magnesium prophylaxis of migraine? Effects on intracellular magnesium," *Headache,* 31 (1991): 298–301.

Fleischauer, A.T., Simonsen, N., Arab, L., "Antioxidant supplements and risk of breast cancer recurrence and breast cancer-related mortality among postmenopausal women," *Nutrition and Cancer,* 46(1) (2003): 15–22.

Frachiewicz, E., et al., "Evaluation and management of premenstrual syndrome and premenstrual syndrome dysphoric disorder," *J Am Pharm Assoc,* 41 (3) (2001): 437–447.

Goldin, B.R., et al., "Estrogen patterns and plasma levels in vegetarian and omnivorous women," *New Engl J Med,* 307 (1982): 1542–1547.

Gorbach, S.L., et al., "Diet and the excretion and enterohepatic cycling of estrogens," *Prev Med,* 16 (1987): 525–531.

Gorlich, N., "Treatment of ovarian disorders in general practice," *Arztl Prax,* 14 (1962): 1742–1743.

Halbreich, U., et al., "Serum-prolactin in women with premenstrual syndrome," *Lancet,* 2 (1976): 654–656.

Heck, A., et al., "Potential interactions between alternative therapies and warfarin," *Am J Health – Syst Pharm,* 57 (13) (2000): 1221–1227.

Horrobin, D.F., "The role of essential fatty acids and prostaglandins in the premenstrual syndrome," *J Reprod Med,* 28 (1983): 465–468.

Hunter, D.J., Manson, J.E., Colditz, G.A., Stampfer, M.J., Rosner, B., et al., "A prospective study of the intake of vitamins C, E, and A and the risk of breast cancer," *New England Journal of Medicine,* 329 (1993): 234–240.

Ishihara, M., "Effect of gamma-oryzanol on serum lipid peroxide levels and climacteric disturbances," *Asia Oceania J Obstet Gynecol,* 10 (1984): 317.

Johnson, S.R., "Premenstrual syndrome therapy," *Clin Obstet Gynecol,* 41 (1998): 405–421.

Jones, D.Y., "Influence of dietary fat on self-reported menstrual symptoms," *Physical Behav,* 40 (1987): 483–487.

Kannel, W.B., et al., "Effect of weight on cardiovascular disease," *American Journal of Clinical Nutrition,* 63 (Suppl) (1996): 419S–422S.

Kaunitz, A.M., M.D., "Use of combination hormone replacement therapy in light of recent data from the Women's Health Initiative," *Medscape Women's Health eJournal,* (July 12, 2002).

Khoo, S.K., Munro, C., Battistutta, D., "Evening primrose oil and treatment of premenstrual syndrome," *Med J Aust,* 153 (1990): 189–192.

Klein, V., Chajès, V., Germain, E., et al, "Low alpha-linolenic acid content of adipose breast tissue is associated with an increased risk of breast cancer," *European Journal of Cancer and European Association for Cancer Research,* 36(3) (February 2000): 335–340.

Kliejnen, J., et al., "Vitamin B_6 in the treatment of premenstrual syndrome—a review," *Br J Obstet Gynaecol,* 97 (1990): 847–852.

Knecht, P., "Role of vitamin E in the prophylaxis of cancer," *Ann Med,* 23 (1991): 3–12.

Kotsopoulos, D., Dalais, F.S., Liang, Y.L., McGrath, B.P., Teede, H.J., "The effects of soy protein containing phytoestrogens on menopausal symptoms in postmenopausal women," *Climacteric,* 3(3) (September 2000): 161–167.

Lemay, A., Poulin, Y., "Oral contraceptives as anti-androgenic treatment of acne," *J Obstet Gynaecol Can,* 24(7) (July 2002): 559–567.

Lew, E.A., et al., "The American Cancer Society Study; Variations in mortality by weight among 750,000 men and women," *J Chronic Dis,* 32 (1979): 563–576.

Liebl, N.A., Butler, L.M., "A chiropractic approach to the treatment of dysmenorrhea," *J Manipulative Physiol Ther,* 13(2) (1990): 101–106.

Limon, L., "Use of alternative medicine in women's health," *Am Pharmaceutical Assoc Annual Meeting APHA,* (2000): 1–5.

Limon, L., "Use of alternative medicine in women's health," *Am Pharmaceutical Assoc Annual Meeting. A Ph A, 2000: Pharmacists Conference Summaries 2000,* Medscape, Inc.

London, R.S., et al., "Effect of a nutritional supplement on premenstrual syndrome in women with PMS: a double-blind longitudinal study," *J Am Cell Nutr.* 10 (1991): 494–499.

London, R.S., et al., "Endocrine parameters and alpha-tocopherol therapy of patients with mammary dysplasia," *Cancer Res,* 41 (1981): 3811–3813.

London, R.S., et al., "The effects of Alpha-Tocopherol on premenstrual symptomatology: a double-blind study. II. Endocrine correlates," *J Am Col Nutr,* 3 (1984): 351–356.

Longcape, C., et al., "The effect of a low fat diet on oestrogen metabolism," *J Clin Endocrinal Metab,* 64 (1987): 1246–1250.

Mackay, H.T., and Evans, A.T., Gynecology and Obstetrics In Current Medical Diagnosis and Treatment, (Tierney, Jr., L.M., et al., editors.) 33rd Annual Revision, 1994, Appleton and Large: 589–590.

Maillard, V., Bougnoux, P., Ferrari, et al, "N-3 and N-6 fatty acids in breast adipose tissue and relative risk of breast cancer in a case-control study in Tours, France," *International Journal of Cancer,* 98(1) (March 1, 2002): 78–83.

Masley, S.C., "Dietary methods to reduce LDL levels," *American Family Physician,* 57(6) (1998): 1299–1306.

McNeil, J.R., "Interactions between herbal and conventional medicines," *Can J CME,* 11(12) (1999): 97–110.

Meltzer, H., "Serotonergic dysfunction in depression," *Br J Psychiatry,* 8 (Suppl) (1989): S25–S31.

Messina, M., "Legumes and soybeans: overview of their nutritional profiles and health effects," *Am J Clin Nutr,* 70 (Suppl) (1999): 439–450.

Moorman, P.G., Ricciuti, M.F., Millikan, R.C., Newman, B., "Vitamin supplement use and breast cancer in a North Carolina population," *Public Health Nutr,* 4 (2001): 821–827.

Munday, M.R., et al., "Correlations between progesterone, oestradiol and aldosterone levels in the premenstrual syndrome" *Clin Endocrinol,* 14 (1981): 1–9.

Murase, Y., et al., "Clinical studies of oral administration of gamma-oryzanol on climacteric complaints and its syndrome," *Obstet Gynecol Prac,* 12 (1963): 147–149.

Murkies, A.L., et al., "Dietary flour supplementation decreases post-menopausal hot flashes: effect of soy and wheat," *Maturitas,* 21 (1995): 189–195.

Murray, M., "Remifemin: answers to some common questions," *Am J Natural Med,* 4(3) (April 1997).

Murray, M., and Pizzorno, J., *Encyclopedia of Natural Medicine* (2nd edition), Prima Publishing, 1998: 730–752.

O'Brien, P.M., et al., "Prolactin levels in the premenstrual syndrome," *Br J Obstet Gyn,* 89 (1982): 306–308.

Osteoporosis Society of Canada, "Clinical practice guidelines for the diagnosis and management of osteoporosis," *CMAJ,* (1996).

Pate, R.R., et al., "Physical activity and public health," *JAMA,* 273(5) (1995): 402–407.

Patter, S.M., et al., "Soy protein and isoflavones: their effects on blood lipids and bone density in postmenopausal women," *Am J Clin Nutr,* 68 (Suppl) (1998): 137–139.

Pearlsetin, T.B., Stone, A.B., "Premenstrual syndrome," *Psychiat Clin North Am,* 21 (1998): 577–590.

Penland, J.G., Johnson, P.E., "Dietary calcium and manganese effects on menstrual cycle symptoms," *Am J Obstet Gynecol,* 168 (1993): 1417–1423.

Pteres-Welte, C., et al., "Menstrual abnormalities and PMS: vitex agnus-castus," *Therapiewache Gynakeol,* 7 (1994): 49–52.

Rapkin, A.J., Edelmuth, E., Chang, L.C., et al., "Whole-blood serotonin in premenstrual syndrome," *Obstet Gynecol,* 70 (1987): 533–537.

Schildge, E., "Essay on the treatment of premenstrual and menopausal mood swings and depressive states," *Rigelh Biol Umsch,* 19(2) (1964): 18–22.

Schmidt, P.J., Nieman, L.K., Danaceau, M.A., et al., "Differential behavioral effects of gonadal steroids in women with and in those without premenstrual syndrome," *N Engl J Med,* 338 (1998): 209–216.

Seidlova-Wuttke, D., Hesse, O., Jarry, H., et al, *Eur J Endocrinol,* 149(4) (October 2003): 351–362.

Sigounas, G., et al., "DL-alpha-tocopherol induces apoptosis in erythroleukemia, prostate and breast cancer cells," *Nutr. Cancer,* 28(1) (1997): 30–35.

Simone, B., *Cancer and Nutrition,* Garden City Park, Avery Publishing Group Inc., 1992: 219–223.

Singh, B.B., Berman, B.M., Simpson, R.L., Annechild, A. "Incidence of premenstrual syndrome and remedy usage: a national probability sample study," *Altern Ther Health Med,* 4(3) (1998): 75–79.

Steege, J.F., et al., "The effects of aerobic exercise on premenstrual symptoms in middle-aged women: a preliminary study." *J Psychosom Res,* 37(2) (1993): 127–133.

Stewart, A., "Clinical and biochemical effects of nutritional supplementation on the premenstrual syndrome," *J Reprod Med,* 32 (1987): 435–441.

Stoll, W., "Phytopharmacon influences atrophic vaginal epithelium: double-blind study—cimicifuga vs. estrogenic substances," *Therapeuticum,* 1 (1987): 23–31.

Stolze, H., "An alternative to treat menopausal complaints," *Gyne,* 3 (1982): 1416.

Surazynski, A., Jarzabek, K., Haczynski, J., et al, "Differential effects of estradiol and raloxifene on collagen biosynthesis in cultured human skin fibroblasts," *Int. J Mol. Med,* 12(5) (November 2003): 803–809.

Tannenbaum, A., "The relationship of body weight to cancer incidence." *Arch Pathol,* 30 (1940): 509.

Taylor, D., Mathew, R.J., Ho, B.T., Weinman, M.L., "Serotonin levels and platelet uptake during premenstrual tension," *Neuropsychobiology,* 12 (1984): 16–18.

Terry, P., Rohan, T.E., Wolk, A., Maehle-Schmidt, M., Magnusson, C., "Fish consumption and breast cancer risk," *Nutrition and Cancer,* 44(1) (2000): 1–6.

Thys-Jacobs, S., Starkey, P., Bernstein, D., Tian, J., "Calcium carbonate and the premenstrual syndrome: effects on premenstrual and menstrual symptoms: premenstrual syndrome study group," *Am J Obstet Gynecol,* 179(2) (1998): 444–452.

Toniolo, et al., "A prospective study of endogenous estrogens and breast cancer in postmenopausal women," *JNCI,* 87(3) (1995): 190–199.

Walker, A.F., De Souza, M.C., Vickers, M.F., et al., "Magnesium supplementation alleviates premenstrual symptoms of fluid retention," *J Women's Health,* 7 (1998): 1155–1157.

Walsh, M.J., Polus, B.I., "A randomized, placebo-controlled clinical trial on the efficacy of chiropractic therapy on premenstrual syndrome," *Journal of Manipulative Physiol Ther,* 22(9) (November–December 1999): 582–585.

Walsh, M.J., Polus, B.I., "The frequency of positive common spinal clinical examination findings in a sample of premenstrual syndrome sufferers," *J Manipulative Physiol Ther,* 22(4) (May 1999): 216–220.

Warnecke, G., "Influencing menopausal symptoms with a phytotherapeutic agent," *Med Welt,* 36 (1985): 871–874.

Wei, H., Saladi, R., Lu, Y., et al, "Isoflavone genistein: photoprotection and clinical implications in dermatology," *Journal of Nutrition,* 133(11) (November 2003): 3811S–3819S.

Woods, M.N., et al., "Low-fat, high fiber diet and serum estrone sulfate in premenopausal women," *Am J Clin Nutr,* 49 (1989): 1179–1183.

Wynn, V., et al., "Tryptophan, depression and steroidal contraception," *J Steroid Biochem,* 6 (1975): 965–970.

Yoshino, G., et al., "Effects of gamma-oryzanol and probucol on hyperlipidemia," *Curr Ther Res,* 45 (1989): 975–982.

Yoshino, G., et al., "Effects of gamma-oryzanol on hyperlipidemic subjects," *Curr Ther Res,* 45 (1989): 543–552.

Yuri, T., Danbara, N., Tsujita-Kyutoku, M., et al, "Dietary docosahexaenoic acid suppresses n-methyl-n-nitrosourea-induced mammary carcinogenesis in rats more effectively than eicosapentaenoic acid," *Nutrition and Cancer,* 45(2) (2003): 211–217.

Zhang, S., Hunter, D.J., Forman, M.R., Rosner, B.A., Speizer, F.E., et al., "Dietary carotenoids and vitamins A, C, and E and the risk of breast cancer," *JNCI,* 91 (1999): 547–556.

Chapter 8

Allison, J.R., "The relation of hydrochloric acid and vitamin B complex deficiency in certain skin diseases," *South Med J,* 38 (1945): 235–241.

Amer, M., et al., "Serum zinc in acne vulgaris," *Int J Dermatol,* 21(8) (October 1982): 481–484.

Andrews, G.C., Post, C.F., Domnkos, A.N., "Seborrheic dermatitis: supplemental treatment with vitamin B_{12}," *NY State Med J,* 50 (1950): 1921–1925.

Araugo, O.E., "Vitamin D therapy in psoriasis," *DICP,* 25(7–8) (July 1991): 835–839.

Ayres, S., Jr., et al., "Acne vulgaris: therapy directed at pathophysiologic defects," *Cutis,* 28(1) (July 1981): 41–42.

Barba, A., Rosa, B., Angelini, G., et al., "Pancreatic exocrine function in rosacea," *Dermatologica,* 165 (1982): 601–606.

Bassett, I.B., et al., "A comparative study of tea-tree oil versus benzoylperoxide in the treatment of acne," *Med J Aust,* 153(8) (October 1990): 455–458.

Bittiner, S.B., et al., "A double-blind, randomized, placebo-controlled trial of fish oil in psoriasis," *Lancet,* 1(8582) (February 1988): 378–380.

Bjorneboe, A., et al., "Effect of n-3 fatty acid supplement to patients with atopic dermatitis," *J Intern Med Suppl,* 225(731) (1989): 233–236.

Bunker, V.W., et al., "Selenium status in disease: the role of selenium as a therapeutic agent," *British Journal of Clinical Practice,* 44(8) (1990): 401–404.

Callaghan, T.J., "The effect of folic acid on seborrheic dermatitis," *Cutis,* 3 (1967): 583–588.

David, T.J., et al., "Low serum zinc in children with atopic eczema," *Br J Dermatol,* 111(5) (November 1984): 597–601.

Dreno, B., et al., "Low doses of zinc gluconate for inflammatory acne," *Acta Derm Venereol,* 68(6) (1989): 541–543.

Farris, G.M, et al., "The effect on atopic dermatitis of supplementation with selenium and vitamin E," *Acta Derm Venereol,* 69(4) (1989): 359–362.

Fiocchi, A., et al., "The efficacy and safety of gamma-linolenic acid in the treatment of infantile atopic dermatitis," *J Int Med Res,* 22(1) (January 1994): 24–32.

Flora, K., et al., "Milk thistle (silybum marianum) for the therapy of liver disease," *Am J Gastroenterol,* 93(2) (1998): 139–143.

Gyorgy, P., "Dietary treatment of scaly desquamative dermatoses of the seborrheic type," *Arch Derm Syph,* 43 (1941): 230–247.

Horrobin, D.F., "Essential fatty acid metabolism and its modification in atopic eczema," *Am J Clin Nutr,* 71(Suppl 1) (January 2000): 367S–372S.

Johnson, L., Eckardt, R., "Rosacea keratitis and conditions with vascularization of the cornea treated with riboflavin," *Arch Ophthamol,* 23 (1940): 899–907.

Keipert, J.A., "Oral use of biotin in seborrheic dermatitis of infancy: a controlled trial," *Med J Aust,* 1 (1976): 584–585.

Kojima, T., et al., "Long-term administration of highly purified eicosapentaenoic acid provides improvement of psoriasis," *Dermatologica,* 182(4) (1991): 225–230.

Lidén, S., "Clinical evaluation in acne," *Acta Derm Venereol Suppl (Stockh),* 89 (January 1980): 47–52.

Majamaa, H., Isolauri, E., "Probiotics: a novel approach in the management of food allergy," *J Allergy Clin Immunol,* 99(2) (February 1997): 179–185.

Messaritakis, J., Kattamis, C., Karabula, C., Matsaniotis, N., "Generalized seborrheic dermatitis: clinical and therapeutic data of 25 patients," *Arch Dis Child,* 50 (1975): 871–874.

Meynadier, J., "Efficacy and safety study of two zinc gluconate regimens in the treatment of inflammatory acne," *Eur J Dermatol,* 10(4) (June 2000): 269–273.

Michaelsson, G., et al., "Erythrocyte glutathione peroxidase activity in acne vulgaris and the effect of selenium and vitamin E treatment," *Acta Derm Venereol,* 64(1) (1984): 9–14.

Michaelsson, G., et al., "Patients with dermatitis herpetiformis, acne, psoriasis and Darier's disease have low epidermal zinc concentrations," *Acta Derm Venereol,* 70(4) (1990): 304–308.

National Rosacea Society, "Coping with rosacea: tips on lifestyle management for rosacea sufferers," Barrington, IL: National Rosacea Society, 1996.

Nisenson, A., "Treatment of seborrheic dermatitis with biotin and vitamin B complex," *J Pediatr,* 81 (1972): 630–631 [letter].

Rosenberg, E.W., Noah, P.W., Skinner, R.B.,Jr., "Microorganisms and psoriasis," *J Natl Med Assoc,* 96(4) (April 1994): 305–310.

Salmi, H., et al., "Effect of silymarin on chemical, functional, and morphological alterations of the liver: a double-blind controlled study," *Scand J Gastroent,* 17 (1982): 517–521.

Schreiner, A.W., Rockwell, E., Vilter, R.W., "A local defect in the metabolism of pyridoxine in the skin of persons with seborrheic dermatitis of the 'sicca' type," *J Invest Derm,* 19 (1952): 95–96.

Serwin, A.B., et al., "Selenium nutritional status and the course of psoriasis," *Pol Merkuriusz Lek,* 6 (May 1999): 263–265.

Shalita, A.R., et al., "Topical nicotinamide compared with clindamycin gel in the treatment of inflammatory acne vulgaris," *Int J Dermatol,* 34(6) (June 1995): 434–437.

Sherertz, E.F., "Acneiform eruption due to "megadose" vitamins B$_6$ and B$_{12}$," *Cutis,* 48 (1991): 119–120.

Staberg, B., et al., "Abnormal vitamin D metabolism in patients with psoriasis," *Acta Derm Venereol,* 67(1) (1987): 65–68.

Thappa, D.M., et al., "Nodulocystic acne: oral gugulipid versus tetracycline," *J Dermatol,* 21(10) (October 1994): 729–731.

Tollesson, A., Frithz, A., "Borage oil, an effective new treatment for infantile seborrheic dermatitis," *Br J Dermatol,* 129 (1993): 95 [letter].

Tollesson, A., Frithz, A., Berg, A., Karlman, G., "Essential fatty acids in infantile seborrheic dermatitis," *J Am Acad Dermatol,* 28 (1993): 957–961.

Tulipan, L., "Acne rosacea: a vitamin B complex deficiency," *Arch Dermatol Syphilol,* 56 (1947): 589.

Valenzuela, A., et al., "Selectivity of silymarin on the increase of the glutathione content in different tissues of the rat," *Planta Medica,* 55 (1989): 1550–1552.

Verma, K.C., "Oral zinc sulphate therapy in acne vulgaris: a double-blind trial," *Acta Derm Venereol,* 60(4) (January 1980): 337–340.

Vienne, M.P., Ochando, N., Borrel, M.T., et al., "Retinaldehyde alleviates rosacea," *Dermatology,* 199 (Suppl 1) (1999): 53–56.

Wahn, U., et al., "Atopic eczema: how to tackle the most common atopic symptom," *Pediatr Allergy Immunol,* 10(Suppl 12) (1999): 19–23.

Index

About the Author

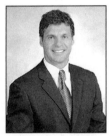

Dr. James Meschino, D.C., M.S., is an associate professor in the division of graduate studies and research at the Canadian Memorial Chiropractic College. He holds a master's degree in science with specialties in nutrition and biology from the University of Bridgeport Connecticut, and has actively taught courses on nutrition and supplementation to naturopaths, medical doctors, chiropractors, estheticians, plastic surgeons, dermatologists, pharmacists, fitness professionals, and the general public since 1984. Dr. Meschino is a frequent speaker at skin-care conferences across North America, where he teaches programs on nutrition, anti-aging, and skin-care management to skin-care professionals.

Dr. Meschino is a post-graduate faculty member of the American Council on Exercise (ACE), and a guest lecturer at the Canadian College of Naturopathic Medicine. He is the coauthor of two wellness books, *The Winning Weigh—7 Steps to Healthier Living* and *Break the Weight-Loss Barrier,* and has had more than seventy nutrition articles published by America Online (AltMed site). He currently writes anti-aging and nutrition columns for a number of professional and consumer publications. Dr. Meschino was a member of the health care staff at the Ryerson University Health Centre, and prior to that ran a private practice in Toronto, Ontario, since 1979. Dr. Meschino is currently the Clinical and Research Director of the RenaiSanté Institute of Integrative Medicine, which provides health care professionals with evidence-based continuing education courses on nutrition and supplementation in anti-aging medicine, disease prevention, and skin-care management.